DR. NOAH VOLZ, DC

THE MASTER STUDENT

BOOK 2

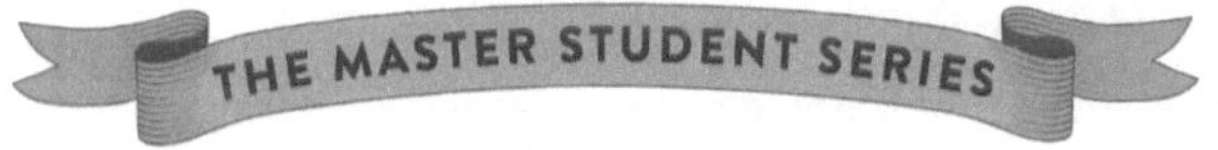

LEARNING

A PRACTICAL GUIDE TO TIME MANAGEMENT, FASTER LEARNING AND GETTING BETTER GRADES IN CHIROPRACTIC COLLEGE

Publishing services provided by:

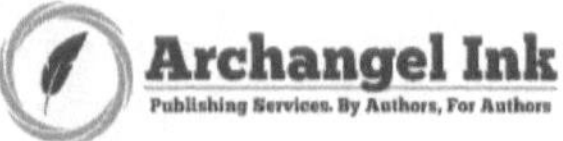

To my family for their continued support. If it weren't for them, I would never have been able to publish this book.

To the millions of students who feel that school is just a hoop they have to jump through instead of a life-changing experience. I hope this book can in some small way make your education more rewarding.

To my teachers, mentors, and coaches. They invested in me, helping me become a better person. Because of their investment, I have something worth sharing.

CONTENTS

Am I a Master Student?

During most of my high school and undergrad years, I thought learning easy—in most subjects, at least. I was never very good at math, but most of my other subjects came easily to me. I could succeed with very little effort. This was back in the nineties before smartphones and laptop computers. More on that in a moment.

When I entered graduate school in 2015, a lot had changed. The classroom environment was completely different than the one I remembered from my undergrad nearly twenty years earlier. The tools I'd used back then seemed to have gone out of style, and I bought into the idea that there was a new way to learn, a better way to learn. To my surprise, I came to see during my three years in graduate school that many of the strategies and tools I used in the nineties hadn't become outdated; they were actually more effective than contemporary methods, allowing me to learn faster and retain more.

At first, I thought my challenges with learning had to

do with my age: I was an adult learner, I was older, and I couldn't pick things up as fast. The truth was that the new style of learning I adopted was at the root of the problem, so I started to study the science behind learning. I explored the different types of memory. I identified how I learn and discovered how most people learn. This book is the result of my research.

While I was in school I had a YouTube channel where I interviewed over one hundred chiropractors. All of them advised listeners to learn as much as they could. I quickly realized that being taught and learning are two very different activities. You can read books, listen to podcasts, and consume a lot of content without ever learning a thing. This was my first insight, and I wanted to know how we integrate knowledge and consolidate it in long-term memory. This book will show you the steps I used to become a master student.

In my first book I advocated for the master student mindset, characterized by focusing your time on a small number of carefully selected and optimized activities that strongly support the things you value. With this approach, you happily miss out on everything else. This mindset is meant to help you curate the tools that deliver massive benefits. Most students focus too much energy on low-value activities that clutter up their time and attention. You must have a mindset that allows you to miss out on the small things and focus instead on the big impact things that will make you a master student. In this book I focus on how to learn so that you will have the time to focus on those high-impact projects.

THE SCIENCE OF LEARNING

The Basics of Learning

I am no expert at learning, that is probably why I decided to investigate the topic. We all know people who seem to have a photographic memory. These are the people who never take notes or who remember what they learned on the first day of class five years later.

I was in school with many of these students. One student named Dylan was that way. Through attentive listening he would master the material. He never took notes, and he rarely studied outside of class. He had developed an in-class strategy that allowed him to retain the important information presented. The truth is, this isn't just a gift of fate—this is a strategy you can learn. In this book, I'll guide you to develop your own strategy for cultivating powerful and effective recall.

I am not an academic or an educational policy professional. That means this book is based on real-life experience, backed up by the latest research. This research was conducted by me, a student who wanted and needed to improve his learning strategy to be successful in school. This book is for all students who, like me, want to be master learners.

Before getting into the specific tactics you can use to learn faster, it's helpful to know the basics of learning. There are three primary ways learning takes place:

1. **Response strengthening.** Most of school is based on response strengthening. When you get a good grade or a right answer on a test that response is strengthened through rewards. The problem with response strengthening is that you orient your learning based on rewards, not on the actual information you're learning. In my opinion, most of what is wrong with organized learning is rooted in response strengthening. As a result, you will have to go against the flow in graduate school to become a master student. You may need to focus on rewards and associations that bolster your creativity and curiosity instead of striving for a certain grade. You must come up with your own rewards and associations. This means prioritizing rewards that are based on what you are learning and the skills you are mastering instead of the grades. At the very least, consider content-based rewards in addition to grades. By doing this you are strengthening your response to learning, which is

different than relying on your grades to motivate your learning.

2. **Information acquisition.** This is what most tests are trying to assess: what you have added to your memory. This is useful in graduate school. Adding information to a passive learner's memory is the essence of information acquisition. The more information we acquire, the more we can do with it. Most of what is considered learning is information acquisition. The challenge with this method is that it rarely tests long-term memory acquisition and problem-solving ability. This book will help you retain what you have learned and integrate it into the new material you are presented with.

3. **Knowledge construction.** This is where the true rigor of learning takes place, through an active process of constructing knowledge. Knowledge is constructed when you put two or more concepts together. It is created when you draw connections and associations between key facts. It is developed when you apply theoretical knowledge to clinical situations. This is the most active of all learning types.

You've no doubt experienced all three learning types. A typical class is based on students sitting in class (information acquisition), taking a test (response strengthening), and completing a class project (knowledge construction). Since every class relies on all three and most teachers use the same principles, I tried to understand why students learn more from some teachers than others. I will clarify that in a later section. Now that we've recognized the three modes of information delivery and reinforcement, it's time to deepen our understanding of how this information is processed.

In school, we rarely have control over how information is delivered, but we can improve the ways information is processed. How a student processes this information determines how much information is retained. The three principles that guide information processing are:

1. **Dual channels.** At this stage in your education, you have probably realized that most of the processing takes place through hearing or seeing information. This is primarily how information is distributed, and your ability to process verbal and visual material is one of the keys to accelerated learning. These channels are separate—that is why they are called dual channels.

You can only process one of these channels at a time.

Since verbal and visual material are separate channels, you want to use both of them efficiently as you study. This was the first element I changed in my learning style. I was used to engaging in the verbal channel as I listened to the teacher while being distracted in the visual channel as I surfed the web on my iPad. If your teacher is not providing adequate visual stimulus to keep those dual channels bringing in information, you'll need to take on that responsibility. This is one of the biggest mistakes students make.

2. **Limited capacity.** Your ability to process information depends on your capacity; everyone has a limited capacity. Through the exercises in this book, you will figure out how much material you can process. First, you need to know that there is a limited amount of material that each channel can process in a given amount of time. Knowing your capacity and finding ways to expand it will increase your processing, but that has limits.

   As you learn, do not exceed the capacity of each of these channels. This principle is harder to measure.

As a long-time meditator, I have noticed that learning capacity is similar to capacity for meditation. The more I meditate, the more my capacity increases. You will know that you have exceeded your capacity when you tune out and stop paying attention. Increase your ability to pay attention for longer periods of time like I have done with meditation. Even though your capacity is limited, it can be increased. The concepts of dual channels and limited capacity refer to passive learning. You are passively taking in information from a book or teacher in both instances.

3. **Active processing.** Active processing is the best way for real learning to take place. Active processing is composed of focusing on relevant material, organizing it, and integrating it with prior knowledge. The *process* is more important than the *result* when it comes to learning. Getting good at focusing on relevant material is the first step. Being able to recognize relevant material allows you to focus on the right things. The next step is to organize the material into a coherent picture. The more coherent the picture, the better you will integrate it with prior knowledge. It is through this

process that learning takes place. The better you can get at that process, the more learning you will experience.

The last principle is more active. By actively processing the information, you turn the passive components into long-term knowledge. That is why case-based learning and problem-based learning are so revered in education. You are applying the concepts that you learned passively and making them more active by solving a problem with that knowledge.

Consider the example of memorizing a phone number. You have probably heard that phone numbers are only seven digits long because they are easier to remember. This is an example of limited capacity. If you write down the number and say it out loud, you are more likely to remember it—an example of dual channels. If you see similarity in the phone number to another number you have already memorized, you can link the two numbers in your mind. If you convert the numbers to letters into a cheesy tagline, you're more likely to remember it. If you visualize pushing in the numbers and see the geometric pattern it creates, you are more likely to remember it. By linking the phone number to something else, to prior knowledge, or to an active process, you're more likely to remember it. Students who can link new information to their prior knowledge can hold more information in their working memory. This is where it all begins. Pay attention to the examples of learning and information processing throughout this book. Using them as a guide, you will optimize your ability to learn. It will not be easy at first. Learning is rigorous, but it is worth the effort.

The first time I learned about dual channels, limited capacity, and active processing they didn't seem actionable. You may feel the same way. Learning about learning is called meta-learning. Like me, you are probably doing enough word association to be able to pass your tests. So why learn about learning? Because with these tools you can prepare for a test in half the time or barely study outside of class. By understanding these principles and utilizing the strategies and tactics presented next, you can optimize your learning to this level.

Learning Mechanics

Learning is like building a house. A house starts with the foundation. The larger the foundation, the larger the house. It's the same with learning: the larger the foundation of prior knowledge, the more learning takes place. If there is not a lot of prior knowledge, then it is harder to link the new information coming in. The prior knowledge provides a framework for you to organize the incoming information.

Back to the house analogy. If you try to build the roof without the walls, it won't work. Similarly, knowledge and long-term memory are constructed in a sequential way. The incoming knowledge elements are selected and organized based on the framework provided by the prior knowledge. As a student selects and organizes the incoming knowledge, they link it to their long-term memory. This linking allows them to store more in their working memory. The working memory is like the job site at the house. Once the foundation and framework have been established, you keep building every day until the entire house has been constructed. If you stop halfway or get distracted by something else, your knowledge will be incomplete and immature. Have you seen those job sites where the crew disappears a quarter of the way through and no measurable progress is taking place? Don't let your mind look like a half-finished subdivision.

It is important to look at working memory a bit deeper because it is one of the primary bottlenecks in learning. Both sensory memory and long-term memory have large capacity. Sensory memory is the architectural plan of the house and long-term memory is the house itself. Anyone can follow a plan to build the house. Once the house is built it's ready to be used. Working memory is the process in between—the daily activities that happen on the job site. The workers' activity is limited to one job at a time. This is like working memory. It can only be engaged in one task at a time, which makes its capacity smaller than the other two.

That is why you must become the project manager of your mind. You must find a way to mentally organize material into a coherent representation that requires less capacity to hold. Like a carpenter building the first room in the house, you must organize your material sequentially. Select the materials needed to build the room and purchase them. Organize the materials and tools you'll need to build the room. Use the tools and supplies in an integrated way with your team to build the room. If you've ever built a house or remodeled a room, you know that the process is never as clear-cut as that. This is the same with learning. Even when you select the relevant words and pictures and organize them into a coherent mental representation and connect them with each other, you must sometimes backtrack because you are missing something.

So, when you are in class, think about the class as a house. Visualize the finished product—what the class is meant to teach you. Identify the foundational knowledge required to build this house of knowledge. As you are in the classroom, organize and select the information in a way that can sequentially build upon your prior knowledge. That is the process of learning. Eventually, you will build an entire city block with all the knowledge you have accumulated in each subject. Many students don't think of the learning process this way and forget why they are in school.

Just as there is more to building a home than the physical walls, there is more to learning than just the process. If you have made your way into a graduate program, chances are you have been learning in an intuitive way for most of your life. You probably feel like you don't need a lot of instruction to improve the process. Or, like me, you know that you can learn faster and have higher retention, so you're ready to understand the learning process more deeply. This is the goal of the strategies and tactics outlined here and used in the second part, where we look at how to use these tools for accelerated learning.

The Eight Tactics of a Master Student

As you read through these tactics, think about which of them you use on a regular basis and put a checkmark next to those tactics. You will need this information for the next part in the book. Maybe you use all of these tactics effectively. Maybe you feel you have room to grow. Maybe you don't use any of them. Maybe you weren't even aware they existed. By exploring these tactics for learning, you can better understand how you learn and then build on that framework.

		Tactics	
1		**Chunking:** Grouping units of info to make them easier to remember	
2		**Errors:** Omitting or acting in a way that yields an unintended result	
3		**Interleaving:** Mixing different types of learning activities	
4		**Transfer:** Application of prior learning to different contexts	
5		**Spacing:** Breaking practice into small sessions with delays in between	
6		**Scaffolding:** Providing the minimum academic support for success	
7		**Retrieval Practice:** Practicing the retrieval of knowledge to promote long-term retention	
8		**Productive Failure:** Intentionally using failure to promote deeper learning	

Tactic 1: Chunking

In my chiropractic college cohort, there were identical twins. One became valedictorian, beating out her sister by a narrow margin. They were experts at utilizing their working memory to master concepts. I didn't really understand how they achieved such amazing results until I learned about chunking.

Our working memory is limited. The better we can use our working memory, the more information we can learn. The human limit is to hold four to five new things in the mind at a time. When working memory is overloaded, your ability to learn is compromised. Here are the most common chunking strategies.[1]

- **Separating:** Phone numbers are a good example of separating. When you separate a long sequence into three smaller sequences it's far easier to memorize. Separating long strings of information into smaller sequences makes them more digestible. Whenever you are learning, find ways to separate larger chunks of information into smaller sequences that you can

---

1 George Miller, "The Magical Number Seven, Plus or Minus Two: Some Limits on Our Capacity for Processing Information," *Psychological Review* 63, no. 2 (1956): 81–97.

memorize.[2]

- **Classifying:** This strategy is good for procedures. If you have a sixteen-step process, divide it into four categories or groups. For example, group a procedure into introduction, exam, discussion, and conclusion. Any time you can group steps into larger categories, it will help with learning.

- **Connecting:** Acronyms are an example of connecting. The brachial plexus is composed of roots, trunks, divisions, cords, and branches. We can simplify this to R, T, D, C, and B. This is an example of connecting. This is how you can store five chunks of information into smaller chunks.

- **Images:** SketchyMedical is a company that takes this to the extreme. Usually we use diagrams, charts, and timelines to chunk information. SketchyMedical creates images that can be used to memorize information.

- **Patterns:** Look for patterns. Repeating patterns of numbers. Similar procedures. Anything that you can find to link a pattern.

---

2 Nelson Cowan, "The Magical Number Four in Short-Term Memory: A Reconsideration of Mental Storage Capacity," *Behavioral and Brain Sciences* 24 (2001): 87–114.

Memory experts use these strategies to build memory palaces. They have learned how to create more elaborate chunks that will be stored in long-term memory. They have become experts in spotting patterns and removing redundancy. They have found ways to compress information into small useful chunks. They know how to consolidate large amounts of data into a simple law or process. They have learned to understand the data in a more fundamental way. That's most often lost with chunking. It's not enough to create cute groups of information; the best chunking helps with improving existing knowledge and increasing the complexity of those chunks.[3]

Tactic 2: Errors

One of the core aspects of learning is identifying and remediating errors. How you correct errors or how you respond to your teacher's error correction will determine whether you embrace difficult challenges or become risk averse.

____

3 Daniel Bor, *The Ravenous Brain: How the New Science of Consciousness Explains Our Insatiable Search for Meaning* (New York: Basic Books, 2012).

There are three types of errors: slips, lapses, and mistakes.[4,5]

Slips are what happens when there is an unintended action. You have the requisite skill or understanding, but you accidentally commit an error when performing a task. The easiest example to understand is misspelling a word that you know how to spell correctly. When this happens, you often self-correct when given the opportunity. Simply by bringing attention to the slip it is corrected.[6]

Lapses are when an action is missed due to a lapse in memory or attention. When a lapse occurs, you have the knowledge or skill to perform the task, but you forget the answer during the test. When you are in a stressful testing environment, you may have a lapse. There are multiple root causes of lapses. One could be memory recall. If this is the case, then more practice is required. The other could be a lapse in attention. This usually requires an environmental change or a way to mitigate the effects of a stressful environment.

---

4 James Reason, *Human Error* (Cambridge: Cambridge University Press, 1990).

5 James Reason, *A Life in Error* (Boca Raton: CRC Press, 2003).

6 Alice Omaggio, *Teaching Language in Context: Proficiency-Oriented Instruction* (Boston: Heinle & Heinle, 1986).

Mistakes happen when the intention is incorrect. A mistake happens when you guess or believe that you know the correct answer but are actually incorrect. Mistakes happen when you have an incorrect understanding or a lack of knowledge about the subject. Mistakes usually point to a larger misunderstanding in the way material was learned and can provide a good opportunity to relearn material.[7]

Tactic 3: Interleaving

Which approach is better to improve your serve? Practicing your tennis serve a thousand times or practicing your tennis serve backhand and forehand? *Blocking* or *massing* is a system of practicing one type of activity repeatedly, such as practicing just the serve. Practicing a set of related activities such as the serve, backhand, and forehand is called *interleaving*; it's usually more effective. In academics, interleaving means solving for different types of related problems. This type of learning is two to three times more effective than

---

7 Roberta Michnick Golinkoff and Kathy Hirsh-Pasek, "To Err is Human, to Reflect (on the Error) is Divine," *Huffington Post,* April 24, 2017, https://www.huffpost.com/entry/to-err-is-human-to-reflec_b_9764374.

solving one kind of problem. [8]

Blocked practice reduces novelty and thereby leads to thoughtless repetition. In blocking, you employ the same problem-solving strategy repeatedly. You eventually go on autopilot and stop learning from your experience. By contrast, interleaving forces you to stay present. It forces you to be able to discriminate between different types of problems and apply an appropriate strategy. This additional mental effort is what makes interleaving so effective as a learning tool; it also makes it challenging to do. The benefits of interleaving are that you get to practice problem discrimination and strategy selection. By improving those meta skills, you learn faster. These skills are essential in medicine. By developing your ability to discriminate between different types of problems and selecting the appropriate strategy, you will not only be a master student, you will indirectly improve your clinical skills. [9]

When employing interleaving as part of your study tactics,

---

8 Nate Kornell and Robert Bjork, "Learning Concepts and Categories: Is Spacing the Enemy of Induction? *Psychological Science* 19, no. 6 (2008), 585–592.

9 Sean HK Kang, "The Benefits of Interleaved Practice for Learning," in *From the Laboratory to the Classroom: Translating Science of Learning for Teachers*, ed. by Jared Cooney Horvath, Jason M. Lodge, and John Hattie (New York: Routledge, 2016), 91–105.

there are a few guidelines to follow:

1. The problems or tasks must be related to each other. Mixing related types of chemistry problems is more effective than mixing chemistry and anatomy problems.
2. Discrimination must be challenging. Discriminating between mammals and plants is not challenging, but discriminating between different types of plants is.
3. Prior knowledge is required to make the discrimination and strategy selection effective.

The main drawback of interleaving is that it is more challenging; therefore, progress can be slower. However, the increases in long-term skill proficiency and memory retention are well worth the additional effort.

Tactic 4: Transfer

Applying concepts learned in the classroom to daily life is called *transfer*. It is our ability to take the anatomy and physiology we learn in school and apply that to the person sitting in front of us. The two types of transfer are *near* and *far*.

Near transfer is when prior learning can be applied to a closely related context. You learn about a disc herniation and then see a patient with a disc herniation confirmed on MRI. Because of the prior learning, you are more able to problem solve the real-life circumstances.

Far transfer is when prior learning can be applied to different contexts, such as transferring knowledge of neurology to the design of a computer programming application. Far transfer is more difficult than near transfer;[10] therefore, it requires cultivation. Far transfer can be cultivated by (1) varying problem types, (2) varying problem-solving methods, and (3) varying learning contexts. These three elements are the primary ways to practice far transfer. Most students practice the same type of problems, use the same type of problem-solving methods, and are exposed to the same type of learning contexts. You will need to break the mold in order to practice far transfer. Since you may not have much control over the type of problems you are asked to solve or the learning context, it is best to focus on your problem-solving methods.

Most people use the same problem-solving method over and over again based on patterns or heuristics that have

---

10 National Research Council, *Education for Life and Work: Developing Transferable Knowledge and Skills in the 21*[st] *Century* (Washington, D.C.: National Academies Press, 2013).

worked for them in the past. A *heuristic* is a simple, efficient rule you use to solve problems when facing complex or incomplete information. Examples of heuristics are:

- A rule of thumb
- Stereotyping
- Profiling
- Common sense

These heuristics are fine for most situations in daily life, but they have limitations when confronted with more complex problems. That is why Jonathan Bendor at Stanford University developed a toolkit approach to solving a problem. Below find the most common cognitive shortcuts that students use to find a solution:

- **Decomposition:** start small and break the overarching problem into smaller pieces
- **Local search:** learn from experience; look for known, similar solutions and adapt them
- **Seriality:** get from A to B; make one small change first then move on to the next
- **Multiple minds:** remember that many hands make

light work; don't work on a problem alone, find out what others think and use them as resources

- **Imitation:** don't reinvent the wheel, find out what other organizations are doing and copy them
- **Recombination:** mix and match; combine a number of different ideas to create a solution

These are examples of varying problem-solving methods; practicing each of these cognitive shortcuts will lead to far transfer. An example of decomposition is that in school you learned that amplitude and mass create force in a spinal adjustment. Decomposition would be figuring out how to measure amplitude and mass. Then you would determine how to vary each component and how that affects the other one. Then you would transfer what you learned into the physical procedure of an adjustment. This is one way to solve the problem of how to adjust.

Far transfer is an effective way to improve learning and to also see how what you are learning is applicable to environments outside of the classroom.[11]

---

11 David Perkins and Gavriel Salomon, "Transfer of Learning," in *International Encyclopedia of Education*, 2nd ed. (Oxford: Pergamon Press, 1994).

Tactic 5: Spacing

Ross, a student in my class, was a master of spacing. At school we had three twenty-minute breaks throughout the day. Ross would take the material he had just learned, identify what he had retained from class, and study what he didn't retain. This approach meant he never had to cram for a test. This is called *spacing*. When comparing studying in one long session (known as *massing*) to practicing in multiple shorter sessions spaced out over time (*spacing*), the second one creates better long-term learning. Cramming for a test will help you pass the test, but it will not result in long-term learning.[12]

If you were to space the five hours you crammed for the test into one-hour segments, you would have better retention of the material. Within this, different spacing gaps have been studied. If you want to remember something for less than six months, then spacing gaps are 20% of that time frame. For example, if you have a test in one week, you need to study every other day. For a test in a month, you need to study every six days. For a test in one year, you need to

---

12 Nicholas Soderstrom and Robert Bjork, "Learning versus Performance: An Integrative Review," *Perspectives on Psychological Science* 10, no. 2 (2015), 176–199.

study once a month. The research on spacing is specific to one fact or skill and so it does not translate well to an entire subject or an entire class. The retention also depends on the type of practice session that is employed. It is unrealistic to remember everything, therefore, it is important to focus these practice sessions on key concepts and foundational skills so that you are prioritizing essential learning.

Tactic 6: Scaffolding

This term is taken from construction. A scaffold is used to support a building until it is strong enough to stand on its own. In education it refers to providing the necessary support until you can independently perform a task. This is not the same as providing feedback. Instead it is identifying the minimum amount of new information you will need to prevent failure. These constraints around the type and amount of new information will help you to be proficient with the material covered and not feel overwhelmed.[13]

This type of scaffolding requires either self-monitoring or monitoring from a tutor or teacher. The monitoring

---

13 Nicholas Soderstrom and Robert Bjork, "Learning versus Performance: An Integrative Review," *Perspectives on Psychological Science* 10, no. 2 (2015), 176–199.

determines whether the material has been learned and then additional information can be introduced. Most learning does not follow a linear path but instead is a collection of related skills or concepts. Because of this you will not progress through clear cut cognitive stages where it is easy to sequence knowledge and developmental stages. That is why monitoring is so important—because it allows you to adjust based on performance.

Scaffolding is primarily used in medical education to ensure that harm is not done. It corresponds to red flags. Scaffolding is rarely used in advanced degree programs. Productive failure is more effective for advanced students and complex topics. A certain amount of scaffolding may be helpful, but too much will impair learning.[14]

Tactic 7: Retrieval Practice

When I decided to go to chiropractic school, I asked my friend who had just finished medical school with a 4.0 GPA for some advice. She told me to use Quizlet. I didn't understand why until I started to learn about retrieval practice. A

---

14 Nam Ju Kim et al., "Problem-Based Learning for Stem Education: Bayesian Meta-Analysis," *Educational Psychology Review* 30, no. 2 (2018), 397–429.

lot of learning can be reduced to retrieval practice. Retrieving and reconstructing knowledge is the best way to learn. It is better than traditional instruction, intensive review, and self-directed study. Retrieving information is best achieved with tests, flashcards, quizzes, and Q&A sessions. Most educational settings emphasize the input and storage of material by pushing it into long-term memory by rereading material, reviewing notes, and relistening to lectures. In comparison to the type of output or retrieval from long-term memory of tests these are ineffective.[15]

By practicing retrieval of information, you improve long-term retention. This happens when you discover what you know and what you don't know. Most students think they understand something, but a test will help them determine if they really know the material. When students recall this information, it roots it in long-term memory. The connections between a given context and the relevant knowledge are improved. That is why incorporating retrieval practice into your studying is so important. Practice tests are one of the best ways for you to learn. Especially when that feedback

---

15 Henry Roediger III and Andrew Butler, "The Critical Role of Retrieval Practice in Long-Term Retention," by *Trends in Cognitive Science* 15, no. 1 (2011), 20–27.

is immediate.[16]

Rote retrieval of facts is only useful for exam preparation. It doesn't show if real learning is taking place. Rich retrieval is the gold standard because it builds knowledge and skills. This is when tests are used to prepare students to synthesize and apply their learning in novel contexts. The rich retrieval practice uses open-ended questions or practical applications that change as the student improves. This is the best type of retrieval practice for building factual knowledge and developing expertise.[17]

Hopefully, your school provides rich retrieval systems. If not, you will have to create your own short answer essay questions or use the suggestions in part two.

Tactic 8: Productive Failure

Nobody likes to fail, but often we learn best from our failures. Learning occurs through success as well, but failure can promote deeper learning when used to understand complex skills and systems. The ability to deal with and learn from

16 Nicholas Soderstrom and Robert Bjork, "Learning versus Performance: An Integrative Review," 176–199.

17 Peter C. Brown, Henry L. Roediger III, and Mark A. McDaniel, *Make It Stick: The Science of Successful Learning* (Cambridge: Belknap Press, 2015).

failure is essential and can be used as a tool for life skills as well. Productive failure can be a tool for learning based on the kind of learning you are doing, what prior knowledge you possess, and the number of possible approaches. Productive failure works best for specific learning outcomes such as developing a specific skill or understanding a specific system.[18]

The complex physical task of chiropractic adjustments is a good example of where failure can be used. That is because learning this skill has many component parts that are interrelated, which allows for multiple approaches to get the same outcome. The best way to encourage learning is to allow students to attempt different aspects of a skill before being instructed; by trying to figure out the components of a task they can learn the task better. Failure at the task or components of the task are followed up with immediate feedback in alternative approaches that may work based on what the student attempted.[19]

Productive failure is different in that it requires students

---

18 Manu Kapur, "Examining Productive Failure, Productive Success, Unproductive Failure, and Unproductive Success in Learning," *Educational Psychologist* 51, no. 2 (2016), 289–299.

19 Aubreen Darabi et al., "Learning From Failure: A Meta-Analysis of the Empirical Studies," *Educational Technology Research and Development* (2018), 1–18.

to have some prior knowledge of the subject and it provides activities that push you beyond your abilities. This activates your prior knowledge and helps you to identify the gaps between what you know and what you need to know to be successful. Immediate feedback that highlights the differences between your attempts and the possible correct approaches will enhance understanding of the skill and what it takes to master it. Failure must be directly correlated to the task difficulty and not unrelated obstacles.

Productive failure works best when students come up with multiple solutions and approaches to a single problem or task. How many ideas they generate and how they use their prior knowledge in crafting those approaches is more important than coming up with the correct approach. Having multiple approaches to attempt allows students to activate prior knowledge and to discover how different aspects of the skill interrelate. The depth of understanding is increased when the subject is approached with creativity. Some skills and concepts are straightforward, and they are not good activities for learning through productive failure. This approach works best on skills that can be done in multiple ways in order to help the student find the way that works best for them.

The Eight Strategies
of a Master Student

Most learning takes place using the eight strategies that will be outlined next. By understanding how and when you use these strategies, you will become more knowledgeable about your learning capacity and you will be able to increase that capacity. These are the strategies that your teachers should be using in the classroom, but now you have the control and can ensure you are learning what you need to. As you read through these different strategies, please notice which ones are familiar to you and which ones you would like to cultivate more of. This information will help you get the most out of this book.

		Strategies	
1		**Creativity:** Generating novel solutions to problems	
2		**Good Decisions:** Making decisions that prepare you for future success	
3		**Metacognition:** Understanding your own thinking	
4		**Depth of Thinking:** Processing to think about content and improve retention	
5		**Progressive Disclosure:** Modulating the difficulty of an experience based on your expertise	
6		**Intelligence:** Being able to comprehend, problem solve, reason, and learn	
7		**Executive Function:** Cultivating mental processes needed for purposeful, goal-oriented behavior	
8		**Motivation:** Being driven to engage in activities	

Strategy 1: Creativity

There are so many subspecialties in chiropractic, and it can be difficult to decide which one really resonates with you. Exposing yourself to all these different techniques can take a lot of time and effort. I realized early on that the subspecialties were an expression of the people in those communities and the founders of those communities. I realized that by interviewing the founder or someone high up in that specialty I could learn more about that technique in an hour with them than by sitting through a twelve-hour workshop. That is partly why I started my podcast; it gave me a chance to learn from a lot of people and evaluate whether their brand of chiropractic was right for me.

Novel expressions of thought and novel solutions to problems are examples of creativity. Creativity is an important aspect of learning just like intelligence and personality. It is considered a psychological construct and it can be cultivated like many of the other traits of master students. Creativity includes problem identification, idea generation, and evaluation. Problem identification is when you correctly identify and frame the right problems that need to be solved and you identify the barriers that need to be overcome to get a solution.[20]

Identifying the problem can be more difficult than it seems. Getting down to the root of the problem is difficult. One strategy is to keep asking why until you get to the root of the problem. For example, the problem may start with "Why do poor people have more back pain?" Because they do not have resources to prevent it. Why don't they have access to those resources? Because the system only offers them drugs as treatment. You continue asking why until you get to the root of the problem. The better the answers are to these questions the better you will get at figuring out the root of the problem.[21]

Idea generation is also important in creativity. This is what is most often associated with creativity. One of my favorite techniques is making lists of ten ideas. They don't have to be good ideas; the goal is to get to ten. Usually the first seven are easy, but it gets way harder after that. When you look at creativity, most of the suggestions are

---

20 Scott G Isaksen, *Frontiers of Creativity Research: Beyond the Basics* (Buffalo: Bearly Limited, 1987), 189–215.

21 Ginamarie Scott, Lyle E. Leritz, and Michael D. Mumford, "The Effectiveness of Creativity Training: A Quantitative Review Creativity Research," *Creativity Research* Journal 16, no. 4 (2004), 361–388.

on idea generation. It is key to evaluate these ideas and how they can solve the specific problem you are trying to solve. It is best to have a third party to evaluate your ideas and help you to come up with the best idea. This feedback and evaluation is best done after idea generation, not in the middle. Group brainstorming is not a good way to produce ideas unless brainstorming happens individually first. The goal of creativity is to generate different ways to achieve goals, solve problems, and express ideas.[22]

Strategy 2: Make Better Decisions

You will make a lot of decisions while in graduate school. Decisions like who to hang out with and what types of clubs to get involved with. Some of those decisions will be based on convenience. You will hang out with the people in your cohort because that is easy. Other decisions will be based on what seems like the best use of your time. The better you understand yourself and your desires the better decisions you will make.

My classmate, Shar, recognized that she performed best

---

22 Sir Ken Robinson, "Do Schools Kill Creativity?" TED, February 2006, https://www.ted.com/talks/sir_ken_robinson_do_schools_kill_creativity?language=en.

under pressure. She would wait until four hours before an exam to study because that would give her the maximum amount of intensity and focus. Other students would try this strategy and would get overwhelmed. She realized that creating constraints and challenges provided her optimal environment for learning; it worked for her.

When it comes to making better decisions, education is limited by daily challenges and real-world constraints. This is a lot like medicine and so we can learn from what works in the medical field. Medicine is evidence based or evidence informed. In practice, this means that people will trade optimal solutions that take time for "good enough" solutions that can be implemented swiftly. In medicine, doctors focus on a set of practices and tools that work; they prioritize mastering those tools. Removing tools that do not work can be more valuable than adding tools that do.

This is sometimes referred to as a heuristic toolbox.[23] It is important for you as a learner to develop an heuristic toolbox and focus 80% of your effort on the practices that will have the biggest effect in your learning, not trying everything and

---

23 Gerd Gigerenzer and Peter Todd, *Simple Heuristics That Make Us Smart* (New York: Oxford University Press, 1999).

seeing what sticks, although conducting field experiments can be helpful. Try one thing in one class and another thing in another, compare the results, and modify practice based on the results. Remember the goal is to induce better actions. It can be easy to use a strategy that doesn't work because it is familiar. To take better actions and make better decisions it is important to stress test your learning strategies. Creating better ways to get knowledge and skills is the key. There is a lot of misinformation out there and so the heuristic tool box can help guide you. You are devoting a lot of your time to in-depth knowledge and complex phenomena, but this may or may not serve you. Streamlining your approach with a focus on the end goal of patient care is necessary.[24] This will be discussed in detail in my next book. To sign up for updates about that book, visit **www.drnoahvolz.com**.

Strategy 3: Metacognition

The two components of metacognition are awareness and monitoring. *Awareness* refers to knowing or being aware of how you learn best. *Monitoring* refers to paying attention to

---

24 Schoar, Antoinette and Datta, Saugato, *The Power of Heuristics*, Ideas42, January 2014.

and controlling your learning to achieve the best results. All the techniques and tactics in this book focus on metacognition and will improve your awareness and control of learning. You will develop the ability to know what learning strategies work for you and to recognize when it is appropriate to use them. All the strategies presented here are based on the scientific approach and these principles.

Metacognitive ability is composed of knowledge, monitoring, and control. *Metacognitive knowledge* is the knowledge you have about thinking, how the brain works, and what study tactics work best for you. This is how you determine what you know and what you do not know. Metacognitive knowledge is how you evaluate your own thinking and determine your biases. It is the development of your metacognitive ability that will allow you to perform twice as well as other students. Most people are not very good at assessing their level of understanding a topic. Most students overestimate their mastery of a subject. The better your metacognitive capacity, the better you will be at knowing what level your understanding is and what you need to increase that understanding. Through an accurate self-assessment of your mastery of a subject you'll be able to increase your learning capacity.[25]

Metacognitive monitoring is usually developed based off feedback. This feedback can be in-person verbal feedback, but it is most often a type of assessment like a test. Tests help students determine how much they know about a subject. Many students perform poorly even when they believe that they know the material and will perform well. It is through effective metacognitive monitoring strategies that students can better self-assess their own learning.[26]

Metacognitive control is the use of both knowledge and monitoring. The knowledge aspect of metacognitive control is where you identify the tools needed for solutions. You must first have knowledge of possible solutions to problems. Then you can monitor how you are using this knowledge as a tool to improve learning. Through combining knowledge and control you can adapt as the situation demands. This adaptation is how learning is improved. Examples of monitoring are self-quizzing and explaining a concept to another student. These tools help to clarify what still needs

---

25 John Flavell, "Metacognition and Cognitive Monitoring: A New Age of Cognitive-Developmental Inquiry," *American Psychologist* 34, no. 10 (1979), 906.

26 John Dunlosky and Janet Metcalfe, *Metacognition* (Los Angeles: Sage Publications, 2008) 200–232.

to be learned. Most students in graduate school do not have explicit knowledge about the different metacognitive strategies, cognitive tasks, and accurate knowledge about themselves. The more you can acquire these skills, the more you will learn.[27]

Strategy 4: Depth of Thinking Improves Retention

In our class we had two standout learners with completely different strategies. Dylan would listen intently and then ask questions after class. He was using his mind to create a depth of thinking about the subject. Kaitlyn would study incessantly. Reviewing her notes, drawing connections to other material, and explaining concepts to others. Both students found ways to develop depth of thinking to improve their retention. They both developed the necessary intensity that is required for retention.

Intensity is the key ingredient in learning. Learning is hard. The better you become at thinking long and hard about the subject matter, the more you will remember. Intensity is defined by how much the information is elaborated as

---

27 Paul Pintrich, "The Role of Metacognitive Knowledge in Learning, Teaching and Assessing," *Theory Into Practice* 41, no. 4 (Autumn 2002), 219–225.

well as its uniqueness, its relevance, and the frequency it is presented.

Examples of elaboration are connecting, explaining, or expanding on learning. Uniqueness is presenting information that is striking or surprising. Relevant information connects to your prior knowledge and builds on that knowledge. Frequency is presenting information repetitively in multiple formats.

Participation does not equal depth of thinking. Merely going through the motions will not result in learning. There must be active processing that takes place. This will take mental energy, so it is important to take breaks when doing this kind of mental processing so that it can be sustained for as long as is needed to really learn a concept or skill. The more you think about something the more likely it is stored. This goes for correct and incorrect information. You will remember what you think about, not just what you wish to remember, and the depth of thought must be adequate for you to remember it.

Strategy 5: Progressive Disclosure

Information presented to students who are not interested or able to process that information is noise. That is where progressive disclosure comes into play. Although progressive disclosure is primarily used in curriculum design and by teachers, it is important for you to understand. By modulating the difficulty and complexity based on a student's ability, they can excel faster.[28]

The goal of this technique is to prevent cognitive overload by presenting layers of information in a progressive manner. It is common in game design, storytelling, instructional design, and physical space design. Many software interfaces have advanced features that can be hidden from novice users. Learning efficiency is primarily based on progressive disclosure. Most education settings do this naturally. They start with high-level facts and then layer the details over time. Journalism also does this by presenting information in order of importance. Information is disclosed to learners as they demonstrate readiness so that it is better received. This reduces the student's frustration and helps them succeed.[29]

Information complexity is inherent in learning, and progressive learning can manage that complexity. The goal is to keep the learning experience at the edge of the learner's

---

28 John Carroll, *The Nurnberg Funnel: Designing Minimalist Instruction for Practical Computer Skill* (Cambridge, MIT Press, 1990).

29 John Carroll and Caroline Carrithers, "Training Wheels in a User Interface," *Communications of the ACM* 27, no. 8 (1984), 800–806.

ability. Learners must demonstrate mastery of problems in small sets to proceed into greater difficulty—keeping complexity low and difficulty high. Once goals are achieved, you can level up to more challenging levels. The ability to modulate the complexity and difficulty in learning is the power of progressive disclosure.[30]

The goal is to focus on the fundamentals and add in detail on demand until the next state is reached and continue to repeat until the concept is mastered.

Strategy 6: Intelligence

Intelligence is defined as the general capability to comprehend, problem solve, and reason. It is the most researched, validated, and measured construct. Probably because of its association with positive lifetime outcomes like career success, health, longevity, and relationships. Most people believe that academic ability is genetically determined, even though that only accounts for 50% of intelligence.

The other 50% can be increased by education. It has been found that for every year a student is in school, they get

---

30 Daniel Hardman, "Progressive Disclosure Everywhere," *Codecraft,* September 16, 2012, https://codecraft.co/2012/09/16/progressive-disclosure-everywhere/.

IQ gains of roughly 1–5 points. This explains why general intelligence has been increasing over the decades. We still don't know exactly how this happens, but we do know that education can expand skills, knowledge, and experience. It can also increase reasoning and problem-solving skills in different contexts resulting in fluid intelligence. The research agrees that intelligence is not fixed. It is also important to understand common myths surrounding intelligence:

1. IQ tests only measure how good you are at taking IQ tests.
2. Listening to Mozart does NOT make people smarter.
3. Brain training games do NOT increase intelligence.
4. There are NOT seven different types of intelligence.
5. There is NO emotional intelligence.

The takeaway? The best way to increase intelligence is through education.

Strategy 7: Executive Function

To succeed in school, you will need to be able to stay focused. The set of mental processes used to concentrate and pay attention is called executive function. This can be cultivated throughout life and will have a direct relationship with your grades. Not only is executive function important for school, it is also important for physical health, mental health, career success, social wellbeing, and psychological wellbeing. Executive function is the foundation of higher order thinking processes of reasoning, problem solving, and planning. The three executive functions that are the most important are working memory, cognitive flexibility, and inhibitory control.[31]

I cover working memory in detail in other sections. To review: working memory acts as a mental chalkboard where new information is temporarily stored and manipulated. The limit of working memory is five new things at a time. It is these chunks of information that can be used for mental problem solving and relating things to existing ideas. A specific strategy for improving working memory does not have a strong basis in research and evidence at this point.

Cognitive flexibility is your ability to adapt to constraints by thinking creatively and changing perspectives based on these constraints. It is helpful for supporting creative pursuits of all kinds by allowing you to consider alternative

---

31 Adele Diamond, "Conclusions about Interventions, Programs, and Approaches for Improving Executive Functions that Appear Justified and Those That, Despite Much Hype, Do Not," *Developmental Neuroscience* 18 (April 2016) 34–48.

approaches, empathizing with others, changing your mind based on new information, and multitasking. The best way to develop cognitive flexibility is by practicing activities that require empathy, critical thinking, and creativity. While reading fiction, you can practice taking the perspective of different characters and understanding their hopes and fears.

Inhibitory control is your ability to control your behavior, attention, and emotions. To learn, it is essential to resist temptation, delay gratification, and override impulsive tendencies. By practicing delayed gratification and delayed responses, you can develop more inhibitory control. Examples are activities like if-then planning, self-discipline, stress reduction, and extended concentration.[32]

Executive function is developed through spending adequate time doing an activity in a way that is focused on getting better at the activity. It's the discipline that produces the benefits. This is easy if the activities students are involved in are interesting and engaging. Executive function often feels dry and serious, but it does not have to be.

---

32 Adele Diamond, "Activities and Programs That Improve Children's Executive Functions," *Current Directions in Psychological Science* 21, no. 5 (2012), 335–341.

Strategy 8: Motivation

Building a house is difficult and it takes a lot of time, just like learning. If the contractor is not motivated by making money to feed his family, the house will never get built. The more we can understand our own motivation behind learning, the more likely we are to use a strategy for learning that is efficient. Motivation can decrease the amount of effort it takes to learn something. Motivation in learning has been divided into five main types:

1. **Interest.** If you are curious about it and interested in it then you are more likely to learn it. The more interested you are, the harder you will work to learn it.

2. **Belief.** You believe that your hard work will pay off. You believe that your investment in school will bear fruit. You believe that you are getting better at something. All these beliefs will help you maintain your motivation.

3. **Attribute the outcome to effort.** You accept that your success or failure is directly linked to how much effort you invest in something. Because of this, you are

motivated to maintain a high level of effort, because if you don't you will fail.

4. **Goal.** You have a very compelling goal, and it is the completion of that goal that motivates you.

5. **Partnership.** Being part of a group and having the social support to maintain motivation. Others are depending on you, so you find the motivation to maintain learning.

If you are not motivated to learn, even the best instructor or the most advanced curriculum will not help you learn. By understanding and using one or more of these motivation strategies, you will be able to learn better. Once you are motivated to learn, you can focus on the other aspects of metacognition.

Motivation is covered in detail later in the book, this will be a brief explanation because of the importance of motivation as a strategy for learning. There are two types of motivation: intrinsic and extrinsic. Intrinsic motivation is when we desire doing certain activities because we find them pleasurable, and extrinsic is where we do them because we are motivated by an external reward. Learning requires intrinsic motivation to be its most effective. Intrinsic motivation is characterized by autonomy, mastery, and purpose. Autonomy gives the student choices on what they learn. Mastery refers to the opportunities students have to improve. Purpose refers to the activities that will make a meaningful difference.[33]

Intrinsic motivation is rarely present in the classroom environment; therefore, some amount of extrinsic rewards must be employed. These rewards work best when they reward learning and not specific outcomes. Rewards for doing homework and reading books is good, while rewards for grades and test results are bad. The best rewards move students toward becoming more intrinsically motivated by providing progressive gains in confidence. Most students expect that they will get A's if they put in a certain amount of time. These are external rewards and do not promote learning as an end in itself, which can do more harm than good.[34]

Relationships also have a powerful impact on motivation.

33 Richard Ryan and Edward Deci, "Intrinsic and Extrinsic Motivations: Classic Definitions and New Directions," *Contemporary Educational Psychology* 25 (2000) 54–67.

34 Sandra Knispel, "The Right Kind of Motivation Comes From You," *Futurity,* June 23, 2017, https://www.futurity.org/self-determination-theory-motivation-1466882-2/.

If the classroom environment is one where teachers and students can actively engage in learning, the students will often excel. Environments that focus too much attention on control and compliance can be demotivating.

Conclusion

These are the tools and tactics you will need to get better grades in school. Chances are, you already employ many of these strategies. You probably identified many of them and learned ways to enhance them. These sixteen components are the foundation you need in order to be a master student. The next chapter will show you how to use many of these tactics in order to accelerate your learning so that you have more time for the things that you love.

PART TWO

ACCELERATED LEARNING

Introduction to Accelerated Learning

Now that you have an idea of the elements of learning. I have two questions for you:

How many hours will it take for you to ace a difficult exam?

Or, more precisely, how many hours must you study to pass a six-hour exam such as Part 1 board exams?

Do you know the answer? Probably not. Like most students, your plan is to take board reviews, which meet for about twenty-four hours total. So, is that how many hours you need to pass? Or do you need more than that?

What if you could study for half as much time and pass? Not by memorizing, but by learning the material. That is the goal of this book. Your time is valuable, so it's important to maximize your study time. We have all known people who speak dozens of languages, coast through triple course loads, and memorize the names of hundreds of people in one afternoon. Well, maybe that last one is a slight exaggeration. Anyway, here we will look at some of the strategies these high achievers use to do this.

There isn't one single tool that you can use to accelerate your learning. Improved learning happens when you learn to efficiently use the strategies and tactics mentioned in the previous section. I have divided this section into assessment, environment, and deliberate practice. Scott Young, Cal Newport, Josh Foer, and others are pioneers in the field of accelerated learning. They have been training individuals to perform techniques that allow them to cut down on their studying by as much as 75% while getting better grades. In the following pages, you will learn the techniques that they use, plus a few others. These techniques are based on the scientific research presented in the first part. I will do my best to connect the dots from the strategies and tactics in part one to these specific strategies as we go.

Assessment

Assessing Your Baseline

Teachers, administrators, and peers are usually the ones assessing you. It is rare for students to effectively self-assess what is working for them when it comes to studying and learning. I briefly introduced metacognition or meta-learning as one of the eight strategies of a master student. In this section, we'll explore the topic a bit deeper. Remember that meta-learning is understanding how you learn. The best students understand how they learn. The best students know when they have learned a concept. The best students know how much studying they will need for a difficult class. In the first part, I introduced the elements of learning so that you could better understand how learning takes place. In this section, I will give you some guidelines on how to figure out how you learn and how long your current strategy takes you in order to master the information. Remember that I am focused on long-term retention, not memorization here.

Before I get into the assessment, let's review metacognition. It is composed of two parts. One is awareness of how you learn best and the next is how you control your learning for the best results. In this section, you are focused on self-awareness of how you learn best.

Do you know how you learn best?

Take a moment and consider the strategies that you use to learn. Memorization? Retrieval practice? Are you good at these strategies? Do they work for you? In my class, we had five students using exceptional learning strategies they had developed over time. Perhaps they had a mentor. Perhaps they developed those strategies unconsciously. Whatever the case, they learned them and you can too!

Metacognitive awareness is usually developed based on outside feedback, but you are going to develop a baseline assessment of the strategies that you use, the time you devote to those strategies, and the results you get with them.[35]

To get where you want to go, take stock of where you are. It works best to do this process on an actual test or quiz. In my first book, I taught you how to master time management. Those techniques are valuable here as well. You have a test coming up with a list of topics you need to know. It is time to figure out what strategies you use to learn the material

---

35 John Dunlosky and Janet Metcalfe, *Metacognition*, 200–232.

and how far these strategies take you. Here is an example.

I have a twenty-question quiz worth 10% of my grade in two weeks. Every time I sit down to study, I note the time on the document I am studying with. For the first hour, I reread the slides. For the second hour, I reread my notes. Then I test my retrieval practice using Quizlet for an hour. I review the concepts from my notes that I missed and retest myself in the last hour. So, in this example I have studied for four hours and used chunking, errors, and retrieval practice.

Now it's your turn.

This will give you your baseline. The more precise you are, the better; but even if you give it an educated guess, it will give you a baseline to work from. You won't know if you are decreasing the amount of time it takes you to study if you don't know how long you normally study for.

Strategies used x Time they are used = Test results

Like an athlete, you need to know your current stats. If you are a marathon runner, you need to know the time you are trying to beat. Without a baseline you cannot measure how much you are improving. The goal is to improve the strategies that are working for you and to reduce the amount of time that you study. Even if you guess at this stage, it is important to have the number of hours you are trying to beat. Now that you know the quantity of time it takes you on average to study and the primary tactics you use, it is time to explore the *quality of your learning*.

		Tactics	
	1	**Chunking:** Grouping units of info to make them easier to remember	
	2	**Errors:** Omitting or acting in a way that yields an unintended result	
	3	**Interleaving:** Mixing different types of learning activities	
	4	**Transfer:** Applying prior learning to different contexts	
	5	**Spacing:** Breaking practice into small sessions with delays in between	
	6	**Scaffolding:** Providing the minimum academic support for success	
	7	**Retrieval Practice:** Practicing the retrieval of knowledge to promote long-term retention	
	8	**Productive Failure:** Intentionally using failure to promote deeper learning	

		Strategies	
	1	**Creativity:** Generating novel solutions to problems	
	2	**Good Decisions:** Making decisions that prepare you for future success	
	3	**Metacognition:** Knowing one's own thinking	
	4	**Depth of Thinking:** Processing to think about content and improve retention	
	5	**Progressive Disclosure:** Modulating the difficulty of an experience based on your expertise	
	6	**Intelligence:** Knowing how to comprehend, problem solve, reason, and learn	
	7	**Executive Function:** Processing needed for purposeful, goal-oriented behavior	
	8	**Motivation:** Driven to engage in activities	

Self-Assessment and Improvement

As we go through the self-assessment it is important to not lose sight of the goal. That is acquiring the valuable skills used to push you in a career direction that has meaning and purpose. Learning will help you get there, but it is a means to an end. You are learning how to learn so that you can excel in your career. Figuring out how much time you spend on preparing for an exam is the first step.

In the next section I will guide you through the next steps, which will hone your ability to concentrate on a small number of powerful skills and eliminate low-grade distraction. Those steps will help you increase the quality of your studying so that you can decrease the number of hours you spend studying. This section is devoted to getting baseline measurements by doing simple assessments. Once you have an idea of your starting point, it will be easier to see the progress you have made.

Intelligence Assessment

Most aptitude tests have the goal of measuring a student's intelligence. Intelligence is defined as the capability to comprehend, problem solve, and reason. Any test has that goal in mind and assumes that high test scores indicate that you have intelligence, or that you have gained the skills necessary to comprehend, problem solve, and reason and that is why you performed well. IQ tests are considered the gold standard when it comes to measuring intelligence. The challenge is that even though intelligence is the most researched, validated, and measured construct, we still don't know exactly how it increases.

How many people do you know who have taken an IQ test? We know that we want to increase our intelligence, but we often don't know what our IQ is. The most used IQ test series is the Wechsler Adult Intelligence Scale (WAIS). Other commonly used tests include the original and updated version of Stanford-Binet, the Woodcock-Johnson Tests of Cognitive Abilities, the Kaufman Assessment Battery for Children, the Cognitive Assessment System, and the Differential Ability Scale. Most of these cost over $1,000. A quick search for free IQ tests returns plenty of results. I would recommend taking one of these free tests to give you a baseline score. Remember that IQ tests only measure how good you are at taking IQ tests. In the absence of any tests that can adequately assess your ability to comprehend, problem solve, and reason this will at least give you a starting point from which to assess yourself.

Heuristic Assessment

As with clinical reasoning and problem solving ability, it's best to measure heuristics in real time. Let's review what a heuristic toolbox is and why knowing yours is important. Heuristics are simple decision strategies that ignore part of the available information, basing decisions on only a few relevant predictors. This is referred to as a heuristic toolbox.[36]

In many clinical decisions there is a list of probabilities and a long algorithm to follow. While this is useful for research in most clinical setting, doctors don't have the time for that; thus, heuristics are developed. Reducing clinical decision making to one or two parameters has better outcomes and reduces decision fatigue. Doctors and other humans cannot foresee the future and cannot know for certain if a diagnosis is correct or if a treatment will cure a patient. Rather, they have to make decisions under uncertainty and often under the constraints of limited time. According to the fast-and-frugal heuristics research program, these decisions can neverthe-less be made successfully because people can rely on a large repertoire of heuristics—an adaptive toolbox—with each heuristic (i.e., each tool) being adapted to a specific

---

36 Gerd Gigerenzer and Peter Todd, *Simple Heuristics That Make Us Smart.*

decision-making environment. By relying on a heuristic that is well adapted to a particular environment, a person can make sound decisions, often based on very little information in little time.

One reason for the surprising performance of heuristics is that they ignore information. As we have explained above, this makes them quicker to execute, easier to understand, and easier to communicate. Instead of learning algorithms, if you learn heuristics for different spine and joint conditions you will make better and faster decisions. You can also apply these heuristics for other decisions in your life. For more information on heuristic decision making in medicine visit **www.drnoahvolz.com**.

It is important for you to develop a heuristic toolbox and focus 80% of your effort on the practices that will have the largest effect on your learning. Typical students try everything to see what sticks. Don't be typical—be extraordinary. That doesn't mean that you don't try some new strategies. Try new strategies, but once you find a strategy that works, spend all your time getting better at that one strategy. For example, you can try one thing in one class and another thing in another, compare the results, and modify based on those results. Remember that the goal is to take better actions. You may be using a strategy that doesn't work because it is familiar. To take better actions and make better decisions it is important to replace learning strategies that don't work with better ones. This is where most students get caught. It takes effort and commitment to break from the familiar and try something new. That is why so few students become exceptional. Creating better ways to get knowledge and skills is the key. There is a lot of misinformation out there and so the heuristic toolbox can help guide you. You are devoting a lot of your time to in-depth knowledge and complex phenomena, but this may or may not serve you. Streamlining your approach with a focus on the end goal of patient care is necessary.[37]

Heuristics for musculoskeletal care are not common. Although there has been some amazing work in stream-lining algorithms for spine care by the Clinical Compass, biopsychosocial model, and primary spine care program, they still require the accumulation of lots of information for clinical reasoning to occur. Assessing a heuristic toolbox is also challenging at this stage. The goal, should you choose

---

37 Antoinette Schoar and Saugato Datta, *The Power of Heuristics*, Ideas 42, January 2014, https://www.ideas42.org/wp-content/uploads/2015/05/ideas42_ The-Power-of-Heuristics-2014-1.pdf.

to accept it, is to determine the least amount of information that you need to determine what is wrong with someone. Here is an example given by one of my mentors, Dr. Dino Pappas, about tight hamstrings.

There are multiple reasons for hamstring tension. Off the top of my head, I put together the following list. I've listed the problem, the assessment, and the "treatment."

1. Neural Tension – SLUMP Test – Mobilize the Sciatic Tract (Sliders, Pin/Strip Techniques, etc.)

2. Core Control (NMS Control) – ASLR – Core Activation & Stability Exercises (Leg Lowering, Planks, Side Planks, Bird Dogs, Reactive Neuromuscular Training, etc.) and then Reassess ASLR

3. True Mobility/Extensibility Problem ("Adhesion") – Check Hamstring Tension in Multiple Positions like Standing Toe Touch, Toe Touch in Step Standing, Seated Toe Touch (True Extensibility will present as decreased/diminished in all positions) – Load the tissue frequently to stimulate histologic reorganization and also consider manual therapies (pin/strip, IASTM, etc.)

4. Kinetic Chain:

    A. Hip Flexor Tension – Check Mod Thomas –
    Mobilize via Manual Methods or Exercises the
    Involved Hip Flexors

    B. Hip Extension Patterning Errors – Prone Hip
    Extension Test – Address relevant deficits with neu-
    romuscular training and relaxation/tension reduction
    methods

5. Lumbar Referral – Check Repeated or Sustained
Movement Testing – Repeat baseline tests for ROM,
strength, etc. after repeated movement testing.

As you can see, getting to the root of the problem is where a heuristic toolbox comes in handy. A set of streamlined questions can determine which of these five things is going on and if there is any overlap between these various causes. Although this section didn't give an assessment per se, I hope it helps you to identify how important developing your heuristic toolbox is in assessment.

Assessing Fear of Failure

In this book and in many others, you have read about how

important it is to fail. The ability to deal with and learn from failure is essential for life; therefore, failure can be used as tool for life skills as well.[38] Remember that one of the tactics mentioned earlier is productive failure. Productive failure is where you have some prior knowledge of the subject and must identify the gaps between what you know and what you need to know to be successful. You may come up with multiple solutions over time to answer this question. The problem I saw in school is that not everyone experiences failure the same. Some people pick themselves up immediately as if nothing happened. Others need days or weeks to reconcile their failure. And depending on the failure, it can take months. I failed Part 3's the first time I took it, and it took time to recover. That is because I didn't know my risk tolerance. I didn't know how failure averse I was at the time. By learning more about myself and my response to failure, I am now able to recover more quickly from failures. Unfortunately, I have not found a validated test that measures this type of resilience. There are a lot of psychological tests that can provide some guidance, but

---

38 Manu Kapur, "Examining Productive Failure, Productive Success, Unproductive Failure, and Unproductive Success in Learning," *Educational Psychologist.*

ultimately you must learn from failure and from how you respond for the best results.

The one I have found the most helpful was developed by Penn State, called the Performance Failure Appraisal Inventory (PFAI). At the time of this writing you can take it here: http://www.personal.psu.edu/dec9/oldweb/lab/reprints/ pfai_man_brf_03a.pdf

Assessing Fear of Errors

Your growth as a student is dependent on your ability to identify and remediate errors. How you correct errors or how you respond to your teacher's error correction will determine whether you embrace difficult challenges or become risk averse.[39,40] I discussed errors earlier and, as with the other elements of this section, the goal is to find an assessment to see how open you are to error remediation. There is not a specific assessment that identifies individuals who are more able to learn from their mistakes. Mistakes happen when the intention is incorrect. A mistake happens when you guess or believe that you know the correct answer but

---

39 James Reason, *Human Error.*

40 James Reason, *A Life in Error.*

are incorrect. Mistakes happen when you have an incorrect understanding or a lack of knowledge about the subject. Mistakes usually point to a larger misunderstanding in the way material was learned and can provide a good opportunity to relearn material.[41] It is important for you to both be able to identify mistakes and to also identify your overall response to making mistakes. Mistakes are much smaller instances of failure and so the assessment is different. The best assessment I have found has been popularized by the psychologist Carol Dweck. In her book *Mindset: The New Psychology of Success*, she identifies traits of individuals that are more able to learn from their mistakes and adapt accordingly. It is good to know if you have a growth mindset as that correlates to your ability to accept errors in school. A growth mindset test could be found at Mindset Works[42] at the time of this writing.

Summary of Assessments

Most schools employ assessments in the form of tests. Some less traditional schools include formative assessments that

---

41 "To Err is Human, to Reflect on the Error is Divine" by Roberta Michnick Golinkoff and Kathy Hirsh-Pasek, *Huffington Post,* April 24, 2017.

42 https://blog.mindsetworks.com/what-s-my-mindset

help students answer the following questions:

Where is the student trying to go?

Where is the student now?

How can the student close the gap?

Additional summative assessments are used by education institutions that include assessments of all the most important learning goals and compare student performance against clear descriptions of what was expected. Both these assessments are outside assessments, and that is why I did not include them in this section. The goal is to develop a self-assessment strategy that adequately gives you a baseline of your skills and tactics so that you can measure your progress toward becoming a master student. Even if you don't take any of these assessments, you will need to spend time figuring out what your baseline is. How can you measure improvement and determine if these tactics work if you don't know where you start? That is the goal of this section, to give you a baseline so that you can measure your progress.

Environment

The second of the three steps in the accelerated learning process is creating a conducive environment and structure for learning to take place. I know what you are thinking: *I am no interior design expert, I'm a medical professional.* You don't need a degree in interior design to learn how to create an external environment that supports your internal environment. What do I mean? I mean the internal state that you bring to your studies can be crafted to give you the best results possible.

Think about test driving a car. You jump in the basic model costing $12,000 and the seats are hard, the speakers are poor, and the overall feel is basic. Then you drive in the deluxe model that goes for $60,000 and you feel differently. The external environment influences your internal environment and vice versa. We have all been in classes where the teacher drones on; no matter how much you want to pay attention, the environment is not conducive to learning. You will need to create the environment that supports you the best. Sometimes this will mean setting up the external setting;

other times it will mean cultivating an internal environment.

There has been a lot written about how the neighborhood you grow up in and the school you go to can influence success. Many Harvard graduates, my brother included, will say that it's more about the network than the education, meaning that you are surrounded by great people and so you push yourself to belong. When focused on being a master student, you can accelerate your learning by creating an internal and external environment that pushes you to do your best work.

I have been teaching yoga for almost two decades, and one thing I've learned is that the goal of all yoga postures is to create peace of mind. You use the external environment to create an internal state that is balanced and focused. I take the same approach in this chapter. Since you won't always have control over the external environment, you can take charge of your internal environment. In this section I will go into more detail about spacing, scaffolding, motivation, and executive function.

Even though this chapter is primarily devoted to the internal environment, it's important to remember that certain external factors are necessary. You can have all the right strategies and tactics, but if you are trying to study while riding your bike, it won't matter how good your strategies are—it's just not the right environment to learn in. Creating the perfect environment has a lot to do with eliminating distractions, maximizing your focus, and maintaining a flow state. Maintaining a flow state is primarily an inside job. Let us begin by looking at the external environment.

A Conducive External Environment

You'll find that certain environmental conditions make it easy for you to enter the flow state, while other conditions make it nearly impossible. These conditions are individual to you and the type of work that you are doing. The process of determining the environment that works best for you may take time. You may have to experiment with different environments.

To begin, choose between public places and private places and see how productive you are in each. Go to a coffee shop and be objective about the amount of work you can accomplish and the amount you are able to retain. Then study for the same amount of time in a private, quiet environment and see how much you accomplish. Determine your preferences. What tasks do you prefer for certain environments? What environments increase creativity? What environments increase concentration? The more you know about what works well for you, the more you can leverage that. Self-awareness is the most powerful tool you have at your disposal when it comes to studying.

To determine if your study space works, consider the following:

1. How much did you accomplish? Number of pages, number of slides, number of words?
2. Take a quiz to determine your retention. Rate your retention on a scale of 1–10 with 1 being poor and 10 being spectacular.
3. How often were you distracted? Estimate the number of times. What did you do when you were distracted?
4. Did you get into a flow state? What aspects of the environment were conducive to that state?

Ultimately, the space you choose will come down to how it feels more so than what it looks like. If you study in a coffee shop, library, room, etc. take a moment and tune in to the energy in the space. Does the space make you feel awake or asleep? Does it make you want to focus on studying or watch a movie? Knowing the effect an environment has on you is key in developing a productive workspace. Write down three words that you associate with your current environment.

Leave your study space for five minutes; when you return, get a fresh impression and repeat the experiment. Without looking at what you wrote down previously, jot down three more words. If the words you wrote down are not conducive to the type of work you want to do then you may need to find a new study space. If you are having a hard time assessing your work environment, get a second opinion. You may not agree with the person you ask, but they will give you a new perspective you can use to evaluate your environment. Or ask to spend time in other people's study environment to get some ideas of what you really like. If it feels right, you will get more done. There is no one-size-fits-all environment. Once you have a good idea of the environment that is the most conducive for your learning, it's time to focus on your internal environment.

A Structured Environment

Breaks are important. Our minds and bodies have a finite capacity to retain and synthesize new information, and that capacity can be increased using breaks. You have probably experienced a time when you could no longer retain new information after studying all night. The problem with spacing is that some people use it to take frequent breaks, which I call distractions; thus, they never get into a flow state where they are synthesizing information. I have been meditating since I was six years old, and the process of spacing reminds me of the first meditation retreat that I went on. I was in college and it was a Vipassana retreat where we would meditate for thirteen hours a day. That is a lot of meditation for a beginner. Over half the group left on the third day of that ten-day retreat. I started to notice all the ways I would get distracted. I started to notice how I would get distracted by the same stuff repeatedly. *I need to buy that, I need to text them, I need to…* You have probably noticed this tendency in yourself as well.

I like the strategy of Paul Jarvis. He says that studying is like driving. You don't look things up and text while you are driving because it is too distracting. When you are studying, you need to act as if you are driving, staying focused on the task at hand for an adequate amount of time. And how much time? Well, I wish there was a perfect amount of time, but I have found this is different for everyone and that you get better at maintaining focus over time. Start with twenty-minute increments. Study for twenty minutes and take a three-minute break. Set a timer for twenty minutes and do not stray from the task at hand for the entire time. No texting, no web surfing, no online shopping. It is best to space these sessions out throughout the day and do a few twenty-minute sessions per subject each day, but this may not be realistic with your schedule. One of the reasons this works so well is that you are most likely to remember the first thing you study and the last thing you study, so in smaller increments of time you remember more.

An Organized Environment

We live in the age of information overload. It can be easy to spend all your time accumulating all the resources you think you will need to study and not actually studying the material. Unfortunately, textbooks were not written to be read, so a lot of the information out there is dry and unengaging. This is probably why you keep searching for a resource that is engaging and will make learning easy. I've got news for you: that resource doesn't exist. Learning is not easy and entertaining. It takes work; your time is better spent reading the materials suggested by your teacher than trying to find better resources. Once you have the resources, it's time to build a scaffold for when you are studying.

A *scaffold* is used to support a building until it is strong enough to stand on its own. In education, the term refers to providing the necessary support until you can independently perform a task. The information provided in your classes is meant to be a scaffold.

Your first task is to methodically learn the information presented by the teacher. Once you integrate and synthesize that information, you can bring in outside resources. Even though I present this as a linear task, learning does not happen in clear developmental stages. That is why it is important to have a system to scaffold knowledge on. It's a framework of sorts. This applies to how you take notes and the digital environment that you create. Have you ever searched your hard drive for something that you were sure was there but couldn't remember how you named it? It's important that you structure information not just for passing the class but for the long term. How you take notes. How you name those notes. Where you store those notes. These are all parts of your scaffolding, and the better organized you are, the more able you will be to integrate and synthesize new information where it is needed.

Maintain Motivation

Motivation in schools is at an all-time low. With all the digital tools that we have at our disposal, it seems like nobody really cares about learning anymore. Most students are just trying to get the easy A and graduate. There have been a lot of scandals involving universities for just this reason. Because we have access to most knowledge through our computers and smartphones, it doesn't seem as necessary to learn the information. So we don't feel motivated. The problem is that you can't make new connections if you don't have enough foundational information, and when you are with a patient, you will not be able to look everything up. You must find enough motivation to learn the material because you will need it in your career.

Motivation is part of your internal environment, and so you must take control of your thoughts and feelings and use them to find your own unique motivation. Motivation is divided into five types, mentioned earlier:

1. Interest
2. Belief
3. Attribute the outcome to effort
4. Goal
5. Partnership

You must use these five motivations for each subject and find one that keeps you motivated to learn the material. The strategies below combine these elements.

Identify a Compelling Motive

If the environment is perfect but you still can't maintain focus and get into a flow state, you may need to look at your internal environment. You will need to find how the subject matter you are learning is personally important to you. When you care about the subject matter, you will be able to sustain the focus and attention necessary to create an environment for learning.

Ask yourself: Why does this task matter to me personally? Is it relevant for someone close to me? How will learning this help others?

It is inevitable that while in school you will be confronted with assignments that seem pointless or stupid. By using the power of your mind, you can find ways in which these tasks can become compelling. It's on you to find a compelling reason to do work you have to do. Pay attention to the stories you are telling yourself. Do these stories help you accomplish the work you need to get done? Do they zap your energy for staying focused? You need to focus your inner resources on finding why assignments are important so that you are more likely to enter a flow state while studying, or at least can maintain your motivation when your energy is low.

Recognize that the work you do not only benefits yourself but others. That is why in school you hear a lot of affirmations about doing great work to help your future patients. Extremes of selfishness and selflessness are not sustainable and will not result in high-quality attention. The task doesn't need to matter enormously, you just need an impact that is valuable enough to keep you on track with your goals and aspirations.

Find a Worthy Challenge

Once you have identified a compelling motive, it's time to get into studying. The overall feeling you are looking for while studying is that of a worthy challenge. Imagine you're in a race—you're way ahead of your competitor, but then they speed up and you're neck and neck. Can you feel the difference? You probably feel more engaged and present when you are racing against a worthy challenger.

When setting up your environment to study, push yourself in order to approach all assignments in a way that puts them at the edge of your skill level and requires you to develop new skills in order to accomplish them. When approaching a task, look at where it falls on a challenge spectrum. This is a scale of 1–10, where 1 is trivially easy and 10 is impossible. The optimal creative range is 5–9 with a 7–8 being ideal. When a task is too easy, you will go into autopilot and will often go through the motions without really learning anything new. If a task is too hard or too complicated, you will fail. Sometimes at this level of the challenge spectrum you may come up with original work, but you will not believe in your abilities because of the difficulty of the task and so you will not have the necessary confidence to continue or to trust your new ideas.

Fortunately, there are ways to modify a task in a way that will adjust the challenge level. The basic structure is to add more constraints to an easy task to make it more challenging. Breaking difficult tasks into smaller chunks reduces the difficulty of the task. The sky's the limit in terms of these constraints. Teaching a classmate or a child is a great way to create constraints. Maybe incorporating Kendrick Lamar song titles into the teaching or into your study guide could be one example. Whatever will make the task simultaneously more interesting and challenging will work.

Rely on Executive Function and the Flow State

The flow state is an extension of your executive function. Getting into the flow state is an indication that you have created the internal and external environment that is most conducive to learning. There is no easy way to describe the flow state, but once you are there you know what it feels like. The flow state is dependent on your ability to concentrate and pay attention. This is called executive function. Executive function is the foundation of higher order thinking processes of reasoning, problem solving, and planning. The more able you are to design systems, processes, and environment where learning takes place and can be easily accessed ten, twenty, thirty years down the road, the more you will be able to use the knowledge you have acquired and paid a lot of money for.

There are three components to developing the internal environment that creates the flow state we are striving for. These are working memory, cognitive flexibility, and inhibitory control. A flow state can arise when you have cultivated all three of these components. Working memory is the dry-erase board of your mind. The new information that you are reading, listening to, or discussing is processed there. You are drawing connections to previous information, you are finding the limitations of your knowledge, and you are focusing on what is important about the new information.

While utilizing your working memory, you will need cognitive flexibility in order to maintain the flow state. Cognitive flexibility allows you to maintain multiple tasks at once. This could be as simple as reading and taking notes, or it could be a more complex set of tasks. In order to maintain the flow state, you will need to be able to switch between different activities smoothly and transfer different types of knowledge from your study materials into your mind. As you do this, you will need the flexibility to determine what new information is valuable and if you need to change your mind about something based on this new information. As you can see, both of these tasks require a lot of focus and intent. You will need to stay really present with the process and go all in.

The last component of the flow state is inhibitory control. As you are learning new information or finding yourself stuck, you will be tempted to do something else. To learn, it is essential to resist temptation, delay gratification, and override impulsive tendencies. A flow state cannot occur if you are unable to stay focused long enough for it to occur. The flow state is not a magical place; it can be cultivated, and the more time you spend in a flow state, the easier it will become to get into the flow state in the future. Its cultivation is well worth the effort because it will make learning fun again and will indirectly feed your motivation. Create a beneficial cycle where you will be excited to learn, feel amazing while learning in a flow state, and thereby learn more than all your classmates.

Summary of Environment

Hopefully you resonate with the idea that an intense study session where retention is high can be called a flow state. Getting into a state of flow while you are studying is the most important thing you can achieve. Then you can use similar strategies to encourage a flow state when you are doing any activity. Every athlete is aware of this state and tries to create rituals that allow them to reach it faster and stay in it longer. It is the same for students as we are trying to be the best performers they can be. Concentration and focus as descriptors of the perfect state of mind do not encourage the level of creativity and insight that the state of flow encourages.

Deliberate Practice

You are nearing the end of this book. I have covered the strategies and tactics that allow learning to happen and then described how you can optimize your self-reflection and environment to maximize those strategies and tactics. In this section, we will take a deep dive into how to utilize everything we have covered so far. This section is called deliberate practice because that is the essence of learning. As the saying goes, "practice makes permanent." So now it is time to find the ways that work best for you to practice. Now it is time to start really accelerating your learning.

The Secret of High Academic Performers

Most students think the following formula is true:

Good Grades = Time Spent

Chances are you believe that to be true as well. You believe that if you study for x number of hours, you will ace this or that exam. This analysis relies solely on the quantity of hours spent, not on the quality of those hours. So, what determines the quality of your studying? I've had the experience where I am feeling really engaged and really present (high quality) versus the experience of feeling tired and distracted (low quality). The product of my studying is very different based on how I'm feeling. Using Cal Newport's lingo, I have chosen to call this qualitative aspect "intensity." Based on this, the real formula for high-performing graduate students is:

Good Grades = Time Spent x Intensity

The key to using this new formula is learning how to develop intensity when you are studying. The more intensity you have when studying, the less time is needed.

I am not much of an athlete, but I do love listening to podcasts by biohackers who are high-performance athletes, and one thing I have learned is that when it comes to fitness there is no better way than high-intensity interval training. Learning is the same. By using the eight strategies and eight tactics introduced in the first part of this book, you can bring more intensity into your learning environment. The more successful you are at that, the faster you will learn.

We all know students who barely crack a book and

consistently get good grades. That is because they can devote a small number of highly intense hours to the material they are wanting to learn. Some of them are exceptional active listeners and rarely do anything more than pay attention in class. Some take amazing notes that keep them engaged and create intensity. Some of them use study groups and feel the pressure of embarrassment and not performing among their peers and this pushes them to remember. All these strategies work. Your goal is to find the one that helps develop *your* ability to create intensity while studying. If one of these strategies does that for you, then use it.

I know what you are thinking. I thought the same thing. *Can intensity really make that big of a difference?* Or, *I'm so exhausted all the time I don't have the energy or mental bandwidth to create intensity.* Yes, intensity will make a huge difference in the amount of time you spend studying so you can use that time to regenerate so you're not tired all the time.

Intensity can and will create huge productivity. I primarily focus on studying in this section, but I have successfully used these strategies to learn psychomotor skills as well. I will introduce you to tools that will help you to engineer intense focus and concentration into your studying and learning. It is more than that—the essence is to be able to put yourself in a state of flow, a state of curiosity and engagement. To get into this state of flow, you will have to learn how to manage your energy, environment, and processes.

What Is Deliberate Practice?

The type of practice we use can help us improve our skills. The most effective type of practice is known as deliberate practice. Any skill can be mastered with sufficient deliberate practice. It would be great if every graduate school program provided the necessary deliberate practice to master the skills of doing a neurological exam and physical exam, but this is rarely the case. Therefore, you must take it upon yourself to learn how to achieve deliberate practice in order to develop and enhance your skills. There are three widely recognized components of deliberate practice:

1. Emphasis on individual skills instead of a whole skill
2. Immediate and specific feedback
3. Progressive difficulty that challenges the student's ability[43]

---

43 Anders Ericsson et al., "The Role of Deliberate Practice in the Acquisition of Expert Performance" *Psychological Review* 100, no. 3, (1993), 363–406.

When learning anything, it is important to practice with these three components in mind.

Let's look at spinal manipulative therapy through this lens as that is the technique most often associated with chiropractors. Step one is emphasis on the components that comprise an ability. For example, this would be the footing, hip position, arm position, hand position, line of drive, etc. that are used to create the ability of adjusting a part of the body. **Complex skills require mastery of each individual component.** This also helps to identify which component is lacking so that effort can be invested to deliberately practice that component. Eventually, these component skills will become automatic; as they do, you don't need to focus so much energy on them, and you can move on to the next component skill that is important.

Each component must be practiced with immediate and specific feedback until each component is mastered. This is especially true when it comes to learning the spinal adjustments used in chiropractic. General advice is not helpful in this context, and it is better to focus on receiving immediate and specific feedback.

In addition to receiving in-person feedback it is important that this feedback includes measuring

performance, monitoring progress, and determining which types of practicing activities are the most effective for you. This is what the best coaches in the world can do. They can give targeted and immediate feedback until the student is able to perform the activity in the right way.

A lot of students lack motivation because they aren't being challenged or they are being overchallenged. Practicing and studying skills that are at the edge of a student's skill level (not too hard, not too easy) is the key. Find the hardest thing that you can do well and progressively increase the difficulty level so that your skills improve consistently. This can do with intensity of practice or frequency of practice. You must keep pushing yourself to do a higher quantity of higher quality practice until you reach a level of mastery that is transferable.[44] The goal is regular, high-quality practice over a long period of time. It would be nice if we could easily quantify the number of hours it takes to master a skill, but every skill and every student is different and so there is no magic number. There must be enough high-quality practice to grow your skills.

____

44 Anders Ericsson and Robert Pool, *Peak: Secrets From the New Science of Expertise* (New York: First Mariner Books, 2017).

How to Learn Faster through Deliberate Practice

There is no better place than graduate school to make you realize how little time you have for the things that matter, and that's why you have a big incentive to learn faster. The students who learn the fastest are also the students with the best career capital because learning quickly is such a highly regarded skill. Thankfully, there is a lot of research on accelerated learning. A lot of that research was cited in the first part of this book. All these tactics and skills can be used to double your efficiency; I will show you how. The most powerful approach to accelerated learning is deliberate practice as it encompasses many of the other skills.

When students think about learning faster, they immediately think about cramming. If you are trying to condense a four-year program into twelve months, it would make sense that you would have to cram, right? Actually, no. Most exams require problem solving and are highly cumulative. Because of this memorizing doesn't work.

Scott Young has condensed multiple four-year programs into twelve months, and he has shared his method online and in his book *Ultralearning*. He developed a method of speeding up the process of understanding the material. We have all had the experience of finally getting a concept or idea permanently. The typical process that a student goes through to get to this insight is to follow lectures, read the book, and grind out practice questions or reread notes. This is a system of sorts, but there is very little focus placed on generating those "aha" moments. There is very little deliberate practice being utilized, and that is what creates "aha" moments.

How these insights are generated are not well understood. That's because we don't really understand the layered nature of learning. So I'll focus on what is well understood. As Scott Young writes in *Ultralearning*, "Getting insights to deepen your understanding largely amounts to two things:"[45]

1. Making connections
2. Debugging errors

Connections are the cornerstone to learning faster. They have big advantages over rote memorization. You will hear more about them later. Connections are made when you find an access point for understanding an idea. One example of making connections would be to use a metaphor. Imagining

---

45 Scott H. Young, *Ultralearning* (New York: HarperCollins, 2019).

the heart being a pump makes it easier to remember how the heart functions. Another example of a connection is finding a relationship between a concept you understand and a new concept. That's why activity-based learning works so well. Connections and insights go hand in hand. The more connections you draw, the more insights you tend to have. Knowing that connections are important is the first step. **The next step is figuring out how to create more connections as you are learning.**

The second way to learn faster is debugging errors. There have been many exams where I have walked into the test having memorized misinformation. Because I did not fully make connections, I did not have a way to reason through my erroneous thinking. Debugging errors is all about identifying the knowledge you're missing or the pieces of the picture that are incomplete. Software companies use the word "debugging" to refer to the process of going through code and finding these errors. Having a system in place to debug your understanding of concepts will help you create the foundation for more connections.

The tools of deep understanding and accelerated learning are that simple. Form accurate connections and debug errors. I will break them out into more detail, but it is really that simple. The more time you spend developing those skills, the quicker you will learn. Let's look at a strategy that uses these skills.

Learning through Connections

Learning through connections is created by developing insight. So, what is insight and how do you encourage it while you are studying? Here are the steps for developing insight into a concept:

1. Handle concepts by creating metaphors and analogies.
2. Remember facts through association first, repetition second.

Create Metaphors and Analogies

Most classes require an understanding of physiology. Once you "get" the big ideas, then it becomes easier to determine what the corresponding facts, terminology, and core concepts are. That is because the best way to remember facts is through association. The more connections you can make between ideas you have mastered or the analogy you are using, the more likely you will be able to remember the idea. Most chiropractic classes in the basic sciences are very factually dense and those facts lend themselves to those connections. This means that repetition in practice questions, mnemonics, or flashcard-style review will have to be a part of your schooling but will not create long-term learning. The key to this strategy is getting good at two things:

1. Using analogies and imagery for *concepts*
2. Using associations to remember *facts*

I love analogies. If you were to spend more time developing your ability to come up with good analogies instead of honing your memorization skills, you would have A's in every class and a vibrant social life. That is why I describe the intensity of learning as a flow state. It requires creativity to develop analogies. If you are finding that a concept is hard to remember, then create a metaphor or analogy in order to help you. This is a skill that can be developed over time. Analogies help you to learn a concept deeply so that you don't have to relearn it in the future. This will allow it to be a solid foundation for concepts learned down the pipeline. Analogies may be difficult to create. So here are some ideas to get you started.

1. Reduce what you are trying to learn into smaller pieces and master each of those smaller pieces.

2. Use the question "Why?" to probe deeper and find patterns.

3. Suggest up to three metaphors that fit the pattern.

4. Use one of the metaphors to explain the idea.

5. Strengthen the metaphor and repeat the process.

At first, this process may feel laborious. As you get better at it, you will be able to do all five steps in less than sixty seconds. Although they have been outlined as distinct steps, you may find yourself doing this automatically without going through each step in a defined way. At first, it may be helpful to make an artistic impression of the metaphor you have chosen. This may take slightly longer, and it is not always necessary. I find it is helpful to write down each step as you go, but you can run through the steps mentally if you prefer. The most important step is to determine a simple example or metaphor that you can use to explain the concept to yourself. Every other step is used to assist in this step. You only need to go through the five-step process when you get struck. These analogies are used to help you understand the core concept. Many times, after the core concept is mastered you may forget the analogy and that is totally fine. The metaphors are scaffolding for understanding the idea and so you don't need to worry about using the same analogy for multiple concepts.

Memorization Is a Last Resort

Memorization is the most ineffective learning tool you have at your disposal. You may have to use it sometimes, I know. All the hard, but ultimately time-saving, insights that you create through connections, associations, and metaphors will increase your long-term retention. Memorization will not lead to reduced study time and better grades. These other tools will. You choose.

Debugging Errors

Before you can successfully debug errors, you must first go through a couple steps. These steps overlap with the previous chapters on deliberate practice and will be familiar to you as part of the mechanics of learning. The three stages are:

1. Coverage
2. Practice
3. Insight

Debugging will happen in the third stage, and it is important to understand the previous two stages to minimize errors in the first place so that you have less debugging to do.

→ Stage One: Coverage

Coverage is the type of work that most students are familiar with. It is the step where you get a general sense of what you need to learn. Coverage includes watching lectures, doing research, reading books or textbooks. Most students believe that this step is the most important and spend all their time on this step. In terms of accelerating your learning, the amount you can learn per unit of time invested is relatively low. You can save a lot of time by speeding up this step and spending more time on the other two steps instead.

One of the big reasons that Scott is a fan of online learning is because you can watch video lectures at 1.5x or 2x the speed. I use a player like VLC,[46] which allows me to watch an entire semester of courses in two days. Another tool that he uses is to take sparse notes while reading and then summarize in writing what you've learned without looking back over the text. Highlighting is like marking something for later

---

46 http://www.videolan.org/vlc/

and encourages a low level of depth, so it is inefficient for real learning. A better approach is to summarize what you have just read to see what you have retained.

→ Stage Two: Practice

Practice problems are important when testing whether you understand a concept and allowing you to go back and learn material that you need to understand more thoroughly. Here are a few suggestions when using practice problems.

Get immediate feedback. If you are not getting immediate feedback, you are hindering your learning. You want to know immediately if the way you are thinking through a problem is correct. That means you must have the correct answer to the problem close at hand. Practicing without feedback or with delayed feedback slows down your learning significantly. I have also found that getting feedback from your peers increases the intensity of the experience and makes you learn faster than just getting immediate feedback from an application like Quizlet.

Use practice problems to your advantage. As mentioned above, practice problems are a common strategy for learning.

Like the classroom, they do facilitate learning, but it is slow and inefficient. Practice problems will develop a level of understanding, but often you are memorizing associations, which is not a mark of true understanding. Like learning in the classroom, practice problems have their place, but they are not very efficient. The best part of practice problems is that they highlight the areas where you need to develop more competence. The other techniques can be used to develop understanding once you've identified where you need to focus. Because of this, practice problems should be used to point out the areas where your coverage is the weakest. Most of your time needs to be spent in the next step, developing insight.

→ Stage Three: Insight

Both coverage and practice are great for getting you to the place where you can clearly identify what you don't understand. Most people recognize this, but they don't recognize how we are wired to tell ourselves that we understand something (when we really don't), or feel confident in a subject (when we probably shouldn't). The insight technique is based on making connections with previous material, creating associations with similar concepts, and facilitating a deeper understanding.

1. Learn by connections, not by memorization.
2. Learn things deeply the first time, don't let confusion compound.

Learn by Connections not Memorization

I learned the most in chiropractic school during my clinical rounds. Why? Because I was learning through connection. By linking the pathology to the patient, I would retain the specifics of the pathology. I could remember the specific tests and the outcomes of those tests more easily than when I was just memorizing the orthopedic tests. Always link concepts to people you know or other information that you have already mastered to create connections.

Learn Things Deeply the First Time

What I see in chiropractic school is that most students go to class and spend their time distracted and then cram before an exam. I agree that class is not always the best place to learn something, but there is a lot of wasted time in this approach. Time is extremely valuable, so you must learn something the first time you approach it. This can sometimes be grueling to work through a concept, but waiting till the end will result in a lot of wasted effort. If you invest time right away to figure out a concept as you encounter it, you will not be building a shaky foundation and you can easily fill in the holes in your knowledge later on.

Deliberate Practice for Tests

Tests! If you are getting your graduate degree in the health sciences then most of your grades are probably based on tests. How you prepare for and perform on those tests determines your grade in that class. The goal here is to decrease the amount of time you spend preparing for the test. It can be helpful to monitor the amount of time you are used to spending currently to determine how well this strategy works for you as you implement it.

I'll use an example. It is your neuroanatomy final exam. You have been going to class and paying attention. You spend twenty minutes at lunch reviewing the notes you took during class and identifying any holes in your knowledge, and now it is time to study for the exam. Normally you spend about seven hours preparing for your final exams, but you only have three and a half hours before the big exam. You have set up a study space that encourages intensity and concentration and you are ready to make the most of the three and a half hours that you have. Based on the time you have, you split your time into two tasks: notes compression and practice exam.

1. Ninety minutes creating a **note compression** of the core concepts. (This involves cramming all the key facts and concepts onto a double-sided piece of paper).
2. Two hours completing and correcting **one practice exam**.

Note Compression

This version of a note compression is probably different than the ones you have done before. In my biochemistry class, we were able to bring a note card full of the information to the final. Unfortunately, I didn't understand how to organize this note card at the time. I just went through my notes and wrote down all the formulas and concepts that I could fit on the card. Although this compressed my notes, it did not serve as a learning tool. There are two ways note compression can be useful. One is to show how much you have retained from class and the other is to solidify that learning.

In order to solidify learning, think of the note compression sheet as a visual representation of the entire class. If you are like most people, you will remember a face but not the name. So the information you put on the notes compression is secondary to how the information is visually represented. Create a note compression that links concepts together. Use analogies, use images, and use colors so that it's easy to picture your note compression in your mind. The more of these you do, the better you will get at organizing it in a way that allows you to retain the ideas that you are trying to learn. Here are some ideas on how to organize your notes compression.

1. **Group related facts together.** Most anatomy classes have a lot of terminology that can be grouped together to assist with remembering to generate associations.

2. **Translate facts into concepts.** Most anatomy classes require you to memorize a list of facts and terminology. Because concepts are so much easier to retain, it is important to turn those facts into concepts that can be used in the metaphor method.

3. **Learn visual memory techniques such as linking, pegging, and vocabulary association.** These are outside the scope of this book, but they are powerful ways to cut down the amount of memorization necessary.

4. **Personalization.** Make it personal, think of situations

or individuals that the information you are learning would be relevant to and learn as if for them.

5. **Concretizing.** Relate unfamiliar knowledge to familiar knowledge.

6. **Anchoring.** Find familiar situations that can be used to learn the new information.

All these techniques can be used during the compression sheet exercise to ensure that you are not just mindlessly copying information from your notes. Everything that goes on your compressions sheet must have a reason for being there and must connect with another concept.

This compression sheet also acts to check the thoroughness of the information being presented and identify if there are any conceptual holes in the presented material. Lastly, it creates a big-picture image of the entire course and links the concepts presented over multiple lectures.

The second way to use a note compression is to see how much you have retained from class. Once you are familiar with creating a note compression, create one from memory. Don't look at your notes or textbooks or anything else and create a note compression. This is a test to see how much of the class material you have retained and how it is organized in your brain. The more you can do from memory, the better. If you cover all the concepts from memory, then it's unlikely you will need much more time studying in this way and it's time to move on to the practice exam.

Practice Exam

For most classes, you can find old exams or exams that test the information that you are learning. The quality of the exam is important in that it addressed most of the concepts that you are required to know for the exam. The practice exam is a safety check. It is meant to show you if you have adequately learned the material. If you score less than 90% on the practice exam, it shows that the intensity and the quality of your note compression is inadequate. If that happens, take a moment and identify what you could have done differently on the note compression. Then find the concepts on your note compression that relate to the questions that you missed on the exam. Do you understand that concept? Is anything missing from your understanding? This is a form of debugging errors. You are trying to understand what was missing from your knowledge, not just memorize the right answer. Again, the goal is synthesizing and consolidating knowledge to get good grades.

The practice exam will help you identify what's missing in your understanding and allow you to go back and learn those concepts. If you have additional time after going back and have access to another practice exam, take that exam. Again, you need to score over 90% in order to prove to yourself that you have sufficient mastery of the concepts in order to excel in the exam. This process trades quantity for quality. You could spend ten hours on memorization of the concepts in the exam or you could spend three to four hours on note compression and practice exams. Both work, but one can make your time and energy more efficient. You choose.

The Feynman Strategy

Perhaps the most well-known technique for accelerated learning was popularized by Nobel Prize winner Richard Feynman. Although his expertise was in physics and you will be using these techniques to master the health sciences, there is a lot that can be learned from his approach. He developed it while struggling with a hard research paper. He ended up meticulously going through all the supporting material until he understood each piece of underlying evidence for the paper he was trying to understand. He kept making associations and connections until he had a deep well of knowledge for his subject. Feynman's technique is deeply steeped in the scientific method and in ceaseless curiosity. If you are the student who is constantly asking why and trying to get to the bottom of things, then this technique will work well for you. Here are two strategies that he popularized.

Get to the Essential Nature

The first aspect of the Feynman Technique is getting to the essential nature of a concept. Physiology by itself is very complicated, not to mention the allied health sciences that support it. Our minds do not deal well with complexity. We often feel overwhelmed by too much complexity or too many unfamiliar words. Humans are not like the textbooks; they reserve the right to have more than one thing wrong with them at a time. When diagnosing a pathology and determining the correct treatment, it is important to simplify things as much as possible. As I write this, I can't help thinking of Dr. House from *House, M.D.* In a way, that is exactly what he does.

How good are you at simplifying complicated concepts? If you are not sure if you have simplified a concept enough then test it by teaching it to someone else. If you can't explain an idea out loud or on paper without confusion or contradiction, then you don't fully understand it. You can't teach something that you haven't learned. One strategy I have heard about for developing this skill is to explain a pathology to a kid. Maybe it's time to volunteer at a children's hospital so you can learn how those pediatricians communicate with their patients. Get back to basics. What are the most likely causes of this pain? What activities is this person involved in that would lead to one of these causes? What other pathologies might this person have that are masking the normal presentation of their primary complaint? What is the essential nature of a problem?

In chiropractic we talk a lot about getting to the root of the problem. That is really the essence of this technique—wading through all the information and exam findings until you can clearly identify the root of the problem. Not getting distracted by the complexity. This can also be used in learning concepts. This is where most physicians stop, but Feynman takes it one step further. After he understands the essential nature of the problem, he tries to understand it with more thoroughness than before.

He does this by questioning his own thinking. This is where he takes the textbook knowledge and questions its validity. He uses these three questions:

What is the simplest explanation?

How can I tell if my explanation is right?

What would validate my explanation?

These are aimed at extracting the essential information. If the explanation cannot be validated or if there is no method by which its "rightness" can be tested, chances are that the explanation is not true or at least can't be scientifically verified. Or maybe you need to come up with your own set of questions. The simplest concepts are easy to validate. Feynman was a master at making things simpler.

Continuous Mastery of New Techniques

This technique, like the last one also relies on intense curiosity. Once the problem had been identified and it had been reduced to its simplest form, Feynman would seek to solve it. As very few of us will find ourselves on the cutting edge of chiropractic research, this strategy may have more value clinically than it does academically. Where it has value academically is with your study habits. If you are tracking and monitoring your study habits for intensity, you can begin to see what is working and what is not working. It is through that recognition that you can start to evolve your techniques and find new approaches. Feynman would continuously try new methods and ways for solving the essential problem that he had identified. He would use strategies outside his field of expertise. He would make connections with seemingly unrelated problems and find their similarities. This was one of his many gifts. How will you embrace the adjacent possible and continuously master new techniques? How will you stay on the edge of your comfort zone so that you are continuously learning and growing? This technique is much harder to teach because it requires a lot of self-reflection. Yet the benefits are well worth the effort.

Getting to the essential nature of a problem and continuously mastering new techniques are both strategies that are useful in chiropractic school. This is the broad concept behind the technique; now let's look at the specifics.

Using the Feynman Technique

The Feynman Technique is to understand the smaller chunks that make up a big idea. By understanding each chunk of information in isolation, you are more able to make connections and increase your understanding.

The technique is simple:

1. Take out a blank piece of paper.

2. At the top write the topic you want to understand.

3. Explain the idea, as if you were teaching it to someone else.

It sounds too simple, doesn't it? The most important step is the one where you explain the idea. That is the whole technique. When you can explain an idea in your own words and in a simple way, you will have mastered the idea. If you can't explain it then you will find the gaps in your knowledge. You will also find out if you are just memorizing the material (i.e., it is not in your own words and it is not simple). By narrowly finding where you don't have full understanding, you are able to selectively research in a way that supports you finding the precise answer. Consider a few variations that Scott uses below.

For Ideas You Don't Get at All

You've tried this technique and it is going nowhere. You are finding that the gap in your knowledge is just too big to cross. One way to work with this is to go through the technique with the book or resource you are learning from.

Meticulously copying both the authors' explanation as you clarify and elaborate on it for yourself. It is a form of the guided Feynman Technique and is extremely useful when you feel like writing out the concept on your own would be impossible.

For Procedures

This is an effective technique for learning orthopedic exams and adjustments. The process is to go through all the steps of the procedure. As you go, explain **what they do and how they execute it**. Carefully explain each part and pay special attention to how they accomplish what they are trying to accomplish and why they are accomplishing that activity. This technique also works well for biochemistry when trying to understand glycolysis or the citric acid cycle.

Checking Your Memory

Now you have a handful of techniques to prove if you have learned what you needed to learn or at least recognize where your gaps may be. Feynman's last technique involves self-testing by being able to finish a description of a topic without referencing the source material. If you can do that, it means you understand the material.

Developing a Deeper Intuition

The Feynman Technique has some additional benefits beyond just developing the first few layers of understanding. It also provides a way for you to drill deeper from a state of understanding to a state of intuition. Intuition in this context means having the insight we talked about earlier where you have an "aha" moment. It is through this process that concepts or ideas stay with you long term. Creating the circumstances for intuition to arise is not easy, but there are some types of learning that usually lead to these insights.

1. **Analogies.** Again? Yes, insights often happen when you recognize an important similarity between an idea you understand and the idea that you are trying to understand. This is the type of insight that is offered by lectures to get you to understand a concept.

2. **Visualizations.** Forming a mental picture, even an absurd one, will often help to take an abstract idea and make it more tangible.

3. **Simplifications.** A big part of the Feynman Technique. If you can't simplify a concept to explain it to a child or a grandmother then you don't really understand it. When you can condense a complex idea into its

simplest parts and articulate it, the ideas will stick longer and faster.

The Feynman Technique is an effective way of encouraging these types of insights. As you are explaining your idea, use some combination of the three methods above. Your own analogies are often better, but if another analogy works for you then use it. Also, if you are learning in a group environment, you may find that other people's insights work well for you too. So not every insight has to be uniquely yours, they just must be powerful enough to help you learn.

Conclusion to Deliberate Practice

A true master of their craft has mastered the tools that they use. A carpenter knows which tool to use for the job at hand. Two different carpenters may use different tools to accomplish the same task in a masterful way. The results are ultimately more important than the method that is used. When it comes to maximizing your learning, you must master the tools that you use. For many, this means a computer, tablet, phone, paper, multicolored pens, fellow students, and on and on. It could also mean the strategies and tactics covered earlier. You need to establish what your tools are and then master them. You will master them by learning to enter a flow state. The flow state is where you have the highest amount of intensity while you are studying.

The more competence you develop with your tools, the easier it is to enter and maintain the flow state. Mastering your tools clears away the doubt of whether what you are doing is working. The more accomplished you become with the individual tools you use to learn, the more you will be able to turn your study materials into long-term memory. I find this is one of the biggest obstacles to entering a flow state. If you are constantly thinking about the low-level action steps, you will not be able to retain the information that you are learning.

Entering and maintaining the state where you efficiently learn and retain is a skill, not a blessing, an accident, or a fluke. That is why so much time was spent in the first part uncovering the science of learning. I wish I could tell you there is one right way to study. There are a lot of aspects of learning, and you will get good at all of them. The more you practice studying these strategies and tactics, the more likely you will be able to experience this state of optimized learning as a regular, perhaps even daily, occurrence. This is true of any psychomotor skill as well. The master craftsman no longer thinks about the mechanics of the movements they are using to do their job. Your job is learning, and so you want to make that job look easy. The goal of self-assessment is to measure your progress as you go.

PART THREE

ACCELERATED LEARNING GUIDE FOR ANATOMY

A Practical Example of Accelerated Learning Techniques

The following material has been adapted from Yan Minis. The best way to learn is through experience, so I am going to take you through learning the bones of the body to give you an example of how accelerated learning techniques can and do work. Instead of relying on rote repetition, we can leverage the science of learning and deep states of focus to memorize all 206 bones of the human body. Here is how.

Memorization

Bones of the Head and Face

Ever wonder why you can remember scenes from a movie but not your homework? It is because movies activate your imagination and allow you to link words to images. That is the goal of memorizing these bones. I will walk you through my process. But remember that you must come up with your own images in order for this to work.

What is the first image that comes to your mind when you think of the word *frontal*? For me it is a woman exposing herself "full frontal" on a busy street. I close my eyes and see that picture with my mind's eye. Now I need to link that imaginary picture to where the frontal bone is located on my forehead, so I imagine myself being distracted by the "full frontal" and hitting my head. The more vivid and involved with my senses—hearing, sight, touch, smell, and taste—the better I will remember it.

Now, you try. Then write down a synopsis of your image next to frontal bone. Do this for each bone and then keep reading. This process will take about forty-five minutes for the entire body the first time. Over time as you develop your imagination, it will go much more quickly. If you come across words that don't stimulate a mental picture, break them down into parts and come up with an image for each part.

→ Skull Bones (8)

- Frontal bone: woman going full frontal on the street, distracting me, causing me to hit my head

- Parietal bone (2): my friend Paris pulling up on the sides of my head to make me taller

- Temporal bone (2): the temp office where I used to get

jobs with everyone's mouth glued shut

- Occipital bone: Aussie: my Australian web developer friends typing on the back of my head

- Sphenoid bone: Sven, the reindeer from the movie *Frozen*, inside my head chattering away

- Ethmoid bone: ethyl alcohol spurting out of my nose and burning

My images could be more vivid, but they work. Remember, the best images are those that you are familiar with. You can create a story to link all the images together: my Aussie friend and Paris are in the temp office where everyone's mouth is glued shut, so they can't respond to the woman going full frontal except to spurt alcohol out of their nostrils that Sven the reindeer comes to lick up. That is my story.

I must admit I am reluctant to keep going because I'm worried that you won't do this exercise. You need the practice, so do it now.

→ Facial bones (14):

- Mandible: a friend called Mandy

- Maxilla (2): Godzilla: I imagine Godzilla walking on where my maxilla bone is and biting my friend Mandy

- Palatine bone (2): palace: I imagine a palace growing out of the roof of my mouth
- Zygomatic bone (2): "zygote" or a cell: I imagine my skin cells dividing grossly where my zygomatic bone is
- Nasal bone (2): this one is easy
- Lacrimal bone (2): lacrosse: I'm playing lacrosse and my eyeballs are goals
- Inferior nasal conchae (2): conch: I imagine a big conch shell up my nose.

→ Middle ears (6):

- Malleus (2): mallet: a big rubber mallet stuck in my ear
- Incus (2): a pot of ink being poured into my ear
- Stapes (2): staple: someone stapling my ear shut

→ Shoulder girdle (4):

- Scapula or shoulder blade (2): blade
- Clavicle or collarbone (2): collar

→ Thorax (25):

- Body of sternum (gladiolus): a happy flower
- Manubrium: Manchester United jersey
- Xiphoid process (1): an x-ray of a phone

- Ribs (2 x 12): easy enough to know the name; no need for a picture here

→ Vertebral column (24):

- Cervical vertebrae (7): circle: ring around your neck, trying to strangle you
- Thoracic vertebrae (12): Norse god Thor throwing his hammer at your back
- Lumbar vertebrae (5): lumberjack hitting your spine

→ Arms (2):

- Humerus (2): Homer Simpson

→ Forearm (4):

- Radius (2): radar ping on my arm
- Ulna (2): Luna Lovegood, a character in the Harry Potter series

→ Carpal (wrist) bones:

- Scaphoid bone (2): scaffolding around a house
- Lunate bone (2): lune (moon in French)
- Triquetrum bone (2): ticket
- Pisiform bone (2): pisiform: pear-shaped: pear

- Trapezium (2): trapeze artist

- Trapezoid bone (2): trapezoid: trapeze robot artist

- Capitate bone (2): decapitate: decapitated bone

- Hamate bone (2): hamster

→ Metacarpals (palm) bones:

- Metacarpal bones (5 × 2): Metallica on the hand

- Proximal phalanges (5 × 2): pipe flange as fingers

- Intermediate phalanges (4 × 2): pipe flange as fingers

- Distal phalanges (5 × 2): pipe flange as fingers

For the phalanges, just remember proximal, intermediate, and distal. No need to create pictures for them.

→ Pelvis (4):

- Sacrum (1): sack of rum

- Coccyx or tailbone (1): tail

- Os coxae or hipbone, comprising the fused ilium, ischium, and pubis (2): coxae: ox with an isle/island (ilium) on its back, with a pair of skis (ischium) and a ruby (pubis)

→ Thighs (2):

- Femur (2): King Julien, the lemur in *Madagascar*

→ Legs (6):

- Patella (2): Nutella

- Tibia (2): Tybalt from *Romeo and Juliet*

- Fibula (2): a kid who lies

→ Tarsal (ankle) bones:

- Calcaneus or heel bone (2): heel

- Talus (2): tallow, beef fat for cooking

- Navicular bone (2): navigation, Google maps

- Medial cuneiform bone (2): cunei means wedge: I think of three blocks of cheese together; this one is on the inside of the foot

- Intermediate cuneiform bone (2): cunei means wedge: I think of three blocks of cheese together; this one is on the middle of the foot

- Lateral cuneiform bone (2): cunei means wedge: I think of three blocks of cheese together; this one is on the outside of the foot

- Cuboid bone (2) : Rubik's cube

→ Feet bones:

- Metatarsal bone (5 x 2): Metallica on the feet
- Proximal phalanges (5 x 2): pipe flange as toes
- Intermediate phalanges (4 x 2): pipe flange as toes
- Distal phalanges (5 x 2): pipe flange as toes

For the phalanges, just remember proximal, intermediate, and distal. No need to create pictures for them.

Revisions

You'll need to do constant revisions or reviews until the images are anchored in your long-term memory. After you have created pictures and written the associations on your pages, go through the images once again. If you are having trouble remembering a picture, try changing it. If you find that you are remembering the picture but not the word, then the association is not strong enough. You need to make the image more vivid or come up with another picture. Focus on the ones you don't know. You'll find that after several reviews there is no need to think of the pictures and come up with the associations. The name of the bone just pops up in your head. This means that your long-term memory has successfully integrated the names and that you now have a solid grasp of the bones in the human body.

Applying Accelerated Learning Techniques to Studying Anatomy

There are three subjects that I consider vital for any doctor: anatomy, physiology, and pathology. Physiology can be learned by understanding concepts and making associations. Pathology can be learned firsthand as you treat patients. Anatomy can be harder to learn, though. Most chiropractic students learn anatomy during their first year and never go back to it again. The techniques in this section will help you learn and retain your anatomical knowledge. Knowing that you have regular reviews of this subject even after four years, will put you at a serious advantage. The best way to keep anatomy fresh in your mind later on during your studies is practical application of what you learned early in anatomy.

Greek Anatomy

Most of medicine is Greek. These tables will help you with the Latin and Greek roots used in anatomy and physiology:

English Form	Meaning	Example
angi(o)–	vessel	angiogram
arthr(o)–	joint	arthritis
bronch–	air passage	bronchitis
calc(i)–	calcium	calcify
card(i)–	heart	cardiovascular
cili–	small hair	cilia
corp–	body	corpus luteum
crani–	skull	cranium
cut(an)–	skin	cutaneous
gastr(o)–	stomach, belly	gastric
hemat(o)–	blood	hematology
hyster(o)–	womb	hysterectomy
lig–	to bind	ligament
osteo–	bone	osteoblast
pleur–	side, rib	pleural cavity
pulm(o)–	lung	pulmonary
ren–	kidney	renal
squam–	scale, flat	squamous
thorac–	chest	thoracic
vasc–	vessel	vascular

Prefixes and Suffixes

English Form	Meaning	Example
a(n)–	without, not	anaerobic
aut(o)–	self	autonomic
dys–	bad, disordered	dysplasia
ec–, ex(o)–, ect–	out, outside	exoskeleton
end(o)–	within, inside, inner	endometrium
epi–	over, above	epidermis
hyper–	excessive, high	hyperextension
hypo–	deficient, below	hypothalamus
inter–	between, among	interoceptor
intra–	within, inside	intraocular
iso–	equal, same	isotope
meta–	beside, after	metacarpus
ortho–	straight, correct	orthopedic
para–	beside, near, alongside	parathyroid
peri–	around	pericardium
sub–	under	subcutaneous
trans–	across, beyond, through	transplant
–blast	to sprout, to make, to bud	chloroblast
–clast	to break, broken	osteoclast
–crine	to release, to secrete	endocrine

Roots

Body part or component	Greek root	Latin root
abdomen	lapar(o)-	abdomin-
aorta	aort(o)-	aort(o)-
arm	brachi(o)-	-
armpit	-	axill-
artery	arteri(o)-	-
back	-	dors-
big toe	-	allic-
bladder	cyst(o)-	vesic(o)-
blood	haemat-, hemat- (haem-, hem-)	sangui-, sanguine-
blood clot	thromb(o)-	-
blood vessel	angi(o)-	vascul-, vas-
body	somat-, som-	corpor-
bone	oste(o)-	ossi
bone marrow, marrow	myel(o)-	medull-
brain	encephal(o)-	cerebr(o)-
breast	mast(o)-	mamm(o)-
chest	steth(o)-	-
cheek	-Zygomatic	bucc-
ear	ot(o)-	aur(i)-
eggs, ova	oo-	ov-

eye	ophthalm(o)-	ocul(o)-
eyelid	blephar(o)-	cili-; palpebr-

face	prosop(o)-	faci(o)-
fallopian tubes	salping(o)-	-
fat, fatty tissue	lip(o)-	adip-
finger	dactyl(o)-	digit-
forehead	-	front(o)-
gallbladder	cholecyst(o)-	fell-
genitals, sexually	haemat-, hemat- (haem-, hem-)	sangui-, sanguine-
undifferentiated	gon(o)-, phall(o)-	-
gland	aden(o)-	-
glans penis or clitoridis	balan(o)-	-
gums	-	gingiv-
hair	trich(o)-	capill-
hand	cheir(o)-, chir(o)-	manu-
head	cephal(o)-	capit(o)-
heart	cardi(o)-	cordi-
hip, hip-joint	-	cox-
horn	cerat(o)-	cornu-
intestine	enter(o)-	-
jaw	gnath(o)-	-
kidney	nephr(o)-	ren-
knee	gon-	genu-
lip	cheil(o)-, chil(o)-	labi(o)-
liver	hepat(o)- (hepatic-)	jecor-
loins, pubic region	episi(o)-	pudend-
lungs	pneumon-	pulmon(i)- (pulmo-)
marrow, bone marrow	myel(o)-	medull-
mind	psych-	ment-

mouth	stomat(o)-	or-
muscle	my(o)-	-
nail	onych(o)-	ungui-
navel	omphal(o)-	umbilic-
neck	trachel(o)-	cervic-
nerve; the nervous	neur(o)-	nerv-

system	-	-
nipple, teat	thele-	papill-, mammill-
nose	rhin(o)-	nas-
ovary	oophor(o)-	ovari(o)-
pelvis	pyel(o)-	pelv(i)-
penis	pe(o)-	-
pupil (of the eye)	cor-, core-, coro-	-
rib	pleur(o)-	cost(o)-
rib cage	thorac(i)-, thorac(o)-	-
shoulder	om(o)-	humer(o)-
sinus	-	sinus-
skin	dermat(o)- (derm-)	cut-, cuticul-
skull	crani(o)-	-
stomach	gastr(o)-	ventr(o)-
testis	orchi(o)-, orchid(o)-	-
throat (upper throat cavity)	pharyng(o)-	-
throat (lower throat)	laryng(o)-	-
thumb	-	pollic-
tooth	odont(o)-	dent(i)-

tongue	gloss-, glott-	lingu(a)-
toe	dactyl(o)-	digit-
tumour	cel-, onc(o)-	tum-
ureter	ureter(o)-	ureter(o)-
urethra	urethr(o)-, urethr(a)-	urethr(o)-, urethr(a)-
urine, urinary system	ur(o)-	urin(o)-
uterine tubes	sarping(o)-	sarping(o)-
uterus	hyster(o)-, metr(o)-	uter(o)-
vagina	colp(o)-	vagin-
vein	phleb(o)-	ven-
vulva	episi(o)-	vulv-
womb	hyster(o)-, metr(o)-	uter(o)-
wrist	carp(o)-	carp(o)-

Conclusion

Now you have all the tools, strategies, and tactics you need to excel not just as a student, but in life. Although the focus of this book has been on helping you become a master student, this is a skill that is used outside of graduate school and in the rest of life. Once you master these tactics and strategies, you will be able to start living the life that you have been dreaming about because many of the most successful people employ these accelerated learning strategies. I hope you have enjoyed this book. If so, please consider sharing it with your friends or leaving a review so that more people can get access to this information. Thank you.

Addendum

There are some additional techniques I came across in my research that did not make it into the body of the book. I have included them here.

Finish Assignments Early

On most college campuses, procrastination is the norm. I have consistently found that high performers at chiropractic school do things differently. By starting a project early, they link their assignments to the things that are most important to them and thereby get a lot more out of it. This strategy is designed to help you do less so you can focus more of your effort on doing a small number of things exceptionally well.

That is the theme of this entire book: quality over quantity. By focusing on a small number of highly important and relevant things, you can produce a low-stress and meaningful student life. One way to do this may be to limit yourself to 12–15 units per semester. This is difficult at chiropractic schools that have a flat fee per quarter, so take that into account when selecting a school. Most chiropractors would advise you to use that time to try everything and go to all the seminars. This is the opposite approach. Consolidate your time and stay focused on a small number of activities. Get good at one or two things with the time you have created by finishing assignments early. Focusing will allow you to develop great mentors who are invested in your success and can open many doors for you.

Even though this message is compelling, there is a lot of cultural and social pressure to do things the opposite way, to overschedule yourself to the maximum. The best students are not those with an overloaded course schedule and nineteen extracurricular activities. The best students are not busier—they are more focused.

Apply to Ten Scholarships a Year

If you want to be a standout student, you must find ways to bring content to the awards and honors section of your resume. Most people, having felt the sting of rejection, are no longer interested in applying for scholarships. What most students don't realize is that scholarships are handed down from an overworked, uninterested administrator who was assigned the unfortunate task of choosing a winner from a depressingly small pool of students, many of whom did not apply correctly. Your odds of winning are high if you apply. Many financial aid departments publish a list of scholarships.

In addition to this, you can contact the financial aid departments of other chiropractic schools, and you can try web-based services like FastWeb[47] and FinAid.[48] You may also want to talk to companies you are interested in working for and see if they want to design a scholarship for you. Then choose ten scholarships a year that fit your abilities, passions, and accomplishments. Mark the deadline and apply when the time is right.

These scholarships and honors tend to grow on each other; the more of those you win, the more you will be eligible for additional scholarships.

Work on a Big Project

Standout students have one thing in common: they go above and beyond. Not necessarily by doing more, but by focusing their energy on something big, something grand, something outside of the norm. They take charge of a project and are always working on it, always making it better, always talking

---

47 https://www.fastweb.com
48 https://finaid.org

about it, and it becomes contagious. The exact scope of your big project is unique to you. It is something that you believe will really make a big impact on the world that you will eventually be a part of. You will gain a lot of skills and insight as you grow in your knowledge of this project, so make sure that you are constantly striving toward something more than the students around you. Go for something big.

Be the Best in the Class Once a Quarter

To stand out and be noticed by your professors, you must hand in one assignment or get a 100% on one test per quarter. You want the professor to remember you and notice that you took their class seriously enough to get one of the best grades they have ever seen. This can often be a jumping off point for mentorship, or it can make it easier when you need a recommendation or some other special treatment. Most tests and assignments are not easily dominated, and it may take a lot of effort to turn heads. Choose a class or content that really excites you. Choose something that you can really learn from and grow from. Focusing on one project a quarter is not that demanding as long as you plan ahead, and the rewards for this effort in the long-term trajectory of your career are tremendous.

Ask One Question Every Lecture

Given the technology we have access to now, one of the most difficult struggles you will face is staying focused during a lecture. The most effective way to stay engaged is to make sure that you ask at least one question every lecture. The easiest way to do this is to prep the night before by reviewing the content that will be covered and to write down a list of possible questions. While in class, make any modifications to your questions based on the professor's material and come up with a meaningful question. This approach will help you stay engaged. It will help you to clarify the material and reinforce your understanding. It will also help you stay alert and engaged. This simple technique will redefine your classroom experience for the better.

Acknowledgments

Thank you to all the chiropractic students who support and share my work.

Thank you to all the doctors who have mentored me on my chiropractic journey so far. Honestly, it has been a struggle and I have considered quitting at least a dozen times. It is through your willingness to support and guide me that I have been able to continue. You know who you are.

Thank you to the amazing team I got to work with on this book. I'm always amazed at how a team of editors and designers can transform a book.

My gratitude goes out to everyone in neuromusculoskeletal medicine and manual therapy who works tirelessly to improve outcomes for those in need. I hope in some small way this book can help the next generation of chiropractors to carry that torch.

About the Author

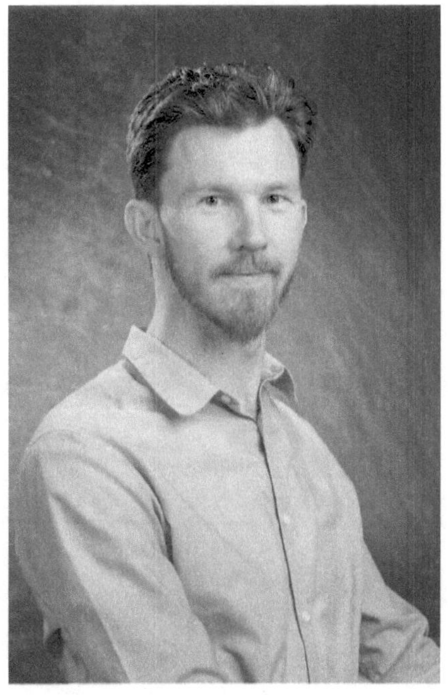

Dr. Noah Volz is an author, chiropractor, and entrepreneur. He has started and run multiple companies and has been the host of the DC2Be Revolution YouTube channel and podcast. Join him at **drnoahvolz.com**.

Connect with Me:

Facebook:

www.facebook.com/drnoahvolz/

YouTube:

https://www.youtube.com/channel/

UCtlEfo4PHGw1hkept5WAw1g

Website:

www.drnoahvolz.com